THE
FIVE
SENSES

THE
FIVE
SENSES

F. Gonzalez-Crussi

HARCOURT BRACE JOVANOVICH,

PUBLISHERS

San Diego   New York   London

HBJ

Requests for permission to make copies of any part of the
work should be mailed to: Copyright and Permissions Department,
Harcourt Brace Jovanovich, Publishers,
Orlando, Florida 32887.

Library of Congress Cataloging-in-Publication Data

Gonzalez-Crussi, F.
The five senses / F. Gonzalez-Crussi.—1st ed.
p.   cm.
ISBN 0-15-131398-9 ✓
1. Senses and sensation.   I. Title.
QP431.G66 1989   88-28966 ✓
612.8–dc19

Designed by Kaelin Chappell
Photographs by Jim Coit
First Edition
Printed in the United States of America
A B C D E

To the memory of Italo Calvino,
who wished to write *The Five Senses*.

Contents

TOUCH

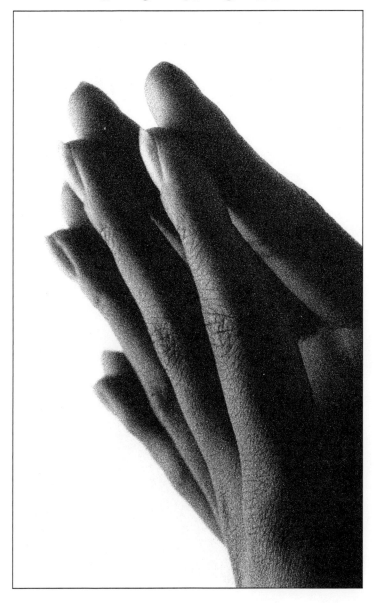

Pain as Riddle

AN OLD GENTLEMAN, a professor of obstetrics and gynecology in my student days, was not above imparting his knowledge with a dash of dubious humor. His wit might have irked a modern apprentice of his art; but I speak of times less harried and more complacent than our own. The secrets of the trade could then bear being wrapped in frolicsome irreverence, and so presented to young pupils, themselves too roguish and too busy to take offense. Thus the professor described the dramatic moments of the birth process with jesting allusions to a "little stranger" who poked his head through a window, looked to one side or the other (which one, it was essential for us to learn: the various rotations of the "presenting head" depend on the sequential engagement of the baby's shoulders and other bodily prominences into the snugly fitting birth canal), then risked sliding out a little farther, and at last, realizing that he (or she) had emerged into a place noisier, colder, filthier, and far more threatening and hostile than his former abode, to which there was no return, uttered a loud wail of frustration and displeasure.

For all its childish ring, this depiction of parturition echoed a widespread notion: that the sanctuary of the maternal womb is the only place on earth where human beings are ever to know the utter bliss of vegetative life. The fetus, it is often assumed, knows nothing of anguish or pain. It exists in an obscure enclosure, wadded up in a posture of hypnotic trance, limbs flexed, bent upon itself. Immersed in a lukewarm fluid that bathes the whole surface of its body, it floats, it buoys with short compassed rotations, moored to the placenta by a pulsating white rope, and attentive only to the rhythmic sibilant rush of the blood flow, and the thumping of another being's heart—another heart, another being, that it cannot yet discern from its own. As this popular version would have it, the onset of delivery marks the rude beginning of a state of sensory stimulation of extraordinary diversity and intensity. Light, sounds, colors, and above all, the infinite sensations conveyed by touch—of which, alas, pain soon triumphs—suddenly assault the newcomer.

This portrayal of prenatal existence is inaccurate. No direct evidence can vouch for the absence of stress and pain before birth, and what little indirect evidence is available would affirm the opposite. It is sad, but inevitable, that this idealized picture of prenatal life should be replaced by a more true-to-life one which leaves room for pain. For we have learned that the late fetus is all but nonsentient. Anxiety and pain seem inseparable from conscious life, even at its early beginnings. Pain, it now appears, is not repulsed by the uterine walls; life's struggle is no less cruel, nor its blows more merciful beneath such lee.

This knowledge did not come easily. Until recent times medical science sanctioned the belief that in early life pain perception is much decreased, or somehow less grievous. There never was a dearth of arguments to buttress the official medical stance, and the case at hand was no exception. The brain of the late fetus and newborn is said to be structurally "unfinished." Many cells persist in it that have not yet reached full development or their final anatomical location. The long fibers that convey nervous impulses, including those registered as pain, are not yet ensheathed in myelin, the structural covering necessary for their integrity and correct function. And is it not obvious that pain is largely psychological in origin? Everyone knows that a mind that anticipates and fears pain is apt to feel more keenly than one untroubled by apprehension and anxiety. Likewise, persons of a stoic temper meet hurtful stimuli more successfully than the maudlin. The newborn infant, whose psychological life is ostensibly rudimentary, was naturally thought to experience pain with less intensity than a more mature, mentally evolved individual. Grandiose hypotheses were not lacking, either: it was proposed that lower sensitivity to pain in the neonate answered to an adaptive purpose, namely, to reduce the stress associated with the process of birth.

The case for giving lesser doses of analgesics to babies undergoing various painful procedures was built upon these premises. On occasion, surgical operations were performed with little or no anesthesia. I hasten to add that valid technical reasons still exist that justify being very cautious about administering strong anesthetics to small, preterm infants (for instance, under the effect of narcotics and anesthetics a small baby may be unusually prone to respiratory depression); but in deciding for or against the use of pain-combating agents, humane considerations did not always carry, in the past, the same importance in newborn as in adult patients. All this changed very recently, when it became clear that the bodily responses associated with pain are uniformly present in the very young. Prematurely born babies, when subjected to painful procedures such as venipuncture, circumcision, or heel lancing, manifest sweaty palms, elevations in blood pressure, increased pulse rate, release of hormones linked to stress, and complex behavioral responses that include altered sleep-wake cycles, irritability, abnormal eye movements during sleep, grimacing, and crying of a type that, when objectively analyzed (as by sound spectral analysis), is seen to correspond to states of hunger, fear, and pain.[1]

That it should have taken a long time for official medicine to acknowledge a phenomenon that at first blush seems obvious is perhaps no coincidence. Pain, like all sense experience, is a private affair. It is fundamentally enigmatic and unknowable. Here we must distinguish between the world of common sense and the realm of philosophical speculation. Medicine, it goes without saying, belongs in the former. In a practical, everyday sense, everyone knows what pain is, and all human beings seem to know when relief is needed. A man tosses about restlessly; his face is pale, and his brow covered with cold sweat; he looks ahead with glazed eyes, and moans most dolefully. Save for perversion, all human beings sincerely pity the man in the grip of pain. Assuredly, pity would not arise in their hearts if they did not believe that his pain is real. It would be ludicrous, perhaps immoral, if the physician's hands were stayed by epistemological cavils. But having once satisfied the moral imperative and the demands of common sense, it is legitimate to wonder, and to speculate. Nay, it is inevitable that we do so. For the stuff of riddles and enigmas is not trapped in the seines of medicine, built for the coarser catch of common sense. But enigmas we need, nonetheless, like daily sustenance.

"Where is the pain?" is a routine clinical inquiry. But "where" is a concept of locality that applies differently in different contexts. Wittgenstein brings home this truth with questions dressed in vivid imagery: "Do we know the place of pain in Euclidean space, so that when we know where we have pain we know how far away from the two walls of this room, and from the floor? When I have pain in the tip of my finger and touch my tooth with it, is my pain now a toothache and a pain in my finger? Certainly in one sense the pain can be said to be located on the tooth. Is the reason why in this case it is wrong to say that I have a toothache that in order to be in the tooth the pain should be one-sixteenth of an inch away from the tip of my finger?"[2] Clearly, there is a sense in which the concept of locality is not the same when we try to define the place of a physical object in space and the place of pain in our body. The geometry of pain is a peculiar one; its orientation and reference points are altogether *sui generis*. The use of coordinates, compasses, or of a grid of intercrossing lines with letters and numbers in them, appropriate for localizing objects in space, seems most odd when applied to pain. Nor is the measurement of distances conceived the same way. For physical objects distances are a matter of objective measurement, and corroboration. But pain perception knows nothing of objectivity; by its very nature it rejects the notion of independent observers. Pain's distances are not metric and objective, but "tactile and kinesthetic."

One does not have a pain in quite the same way as one has a car, or a new dress. For Wittgenstein, to have a pain is to correlate various tactile, sensory, and kinesthetic perceptions. Imagine, to paraphrase his example, the pain of renal colic. The sufferer is conscious of a focus of lancinating pain. He applies his hand against the painful area and feels, all around it, a dull environment of numbness. He has also the tactile sensation against the pressuring hand. And the whole is yet correlated with other perceptions, such as visual ones: the sight of the hand coming to press against the flank, or watching himself doing this in a mirror. If the pain is excruciating, as renal colic often is, there will be other sensations to correlate: the body becoming rigid, the hand coming to rest against the flank, the mouth going dry, the respiratory movements stopping, and the muscles of the painful area involuntarily contracting. Now imagine for a moment that the patient is sitting side by side with other men, in the dark. He experiences an attack of colic, which is to say he experiences all the tactile, visual, and kinesthetic sensations described above together with pain, including those normally bound up with moving his hand toward his aching flank. At this time, however, the lights of the room are turned on, and he discovers that his hand is not pressed against his own flank, but on his neighbor's. The conclusion would have to be that the man "has a renal colic in another person's kidney."

This example is by no means idle. Real life offers paradoxes even more astonishing. Such is the often-quoted example of "phantom limbs" in amputees. The limb has been severed above the knee, but the patient distinctly experiences pain below the amputation site—say, in his foot. But there is no such foot. Thus it may be said, without exaggeration, that the amputee has a pain the location of which is "in an empty space." If I happen to be sitting in close proximity to the patient's stump, it is conceivable that he might trace the location of his pain to my knee or my foot. Is it then correct to say that he experiences a knee ache in my knee? Note, moreover, that if we agree with Wittgenstein that "to have a pain" is to correlate a series of tactile, sensory, and kinesthetic experiences with one another, at least it can be said that these experiences presuppose the existence of the respective anatomical substratum: there *is* a kidney that aches; there *is* a hand that presses against the flank; and so on.

The real-life example of a phantom limb is still more para-doxical and disconcerting, since the limb does not exist at all. It matters little what technical/medical explanations may be offered to "explain" the abnormal sensation (for instance, that abnormal nerve growth at the stump gives rise to perceptible nervous impulses); the fact remains that the amputee feels, with extraordinary vividness, a limb that has no objective reality. The bearer of a phantom limb reports detailed sensations of pain, itch, numbness, dryness, weight, and the like. The toes or fingers and the joints are felt with keenest precision. The patient some-times has the distinct impression that he can actually move the phantom, or else that the limb is in an uncomfortable position, with the toes or fingers curling into the flesh. Amazing as it sounds, this phenomenon illustrates the fact that reality does not have to exist to be perceived: *existence is not a precondition for perception*.

The participation of psychological factors increases the com-plexity of this phenomenon. It is universally agreed that the psychological constitution of the amputee has much to do with the life of the phantom. Emotions and their upheavals may be accountable for the appearance of a phantom limb in an amputee who previously had none. "Ghost" limbs have appeared months or years, up to twenty years, after the amputation.[3] Conversely, the phantom limb may shrink and be progressively "absorbed," as it were, into the stump. Psychiatrists have pointed out that this is likelier to happen in coincidence with the patient's "acceptance" of his mutilation. But if we were tempted to at-tribute the origin of the phenomenon entirely to psychological factors, we would most certainly be in the wrong, since vari-ous surgical procedures and manipulations of the nerves can remove the pain (but often not the sensation) of a phantom limb.

It is a cliché in the medical literature, when referring to such puzzles, to say that "both psychological and organic features interact to produce the symptoms." But textbook statements of this sort explain nothing, and content only the smug or the unthinking. For it is obvious that the whole crux of the problem resides in knowing precisely *how* psychological and organic or physiological factors relate to one another, how they dovetail into each other to produce the observed effect. I, for one, find it incomprehensible that two determining factors, each belonging to a completely different order of things, should mutually interact as if they were of the same nature. I have no difficulty in understanding how a mechanical force working in one direction may be modified by another force exerted in a different direction, and thus give rise to a vector that is, in a concrete sense, the product of the algebraic sum of the other two. After all, only mechanical forces enter into the equation. But it utterly surpasses my comprehension to be told that emotional factors and physical factors combine with each other, or add one to another, to produce a consistent result. How can it be that elements so disparate become articulated in a stable, intelligible fashion? How can it be that nervous impulses, which are physiochemical reactions that take place in the nerves, should dovetail with memories of childhood, fear of death, and all sorts of anxieties and volitions, which reside we know not where, and perhaps nowhere?

But if we were to consider only one aspect of the problem, we would be no less baffled. For how should the psychology of the phantom limb be classified? Is it a case of remembering, since it is a conscious representation of the body as it was, before the mutilation? Or is it an instance of forgetting, since the representation blatantly overlooks the new bodily state, which calls for the suppression of one of its parts? Or is it perhaps a form of volition, since the body is represented as the patient wills it to be? It is none of those things. It is not a memory: the patient does not evoke its presence as he would the thought of a departed friend, or a dead mother. It is not an image conjured up from the past and recast in the bittersweet idealization that memories are wont to assume. But it is not forgetfulness, either: the forgotten is absent from consciousness, whereas the phantom limb is a constant presence. Nor does it seem to be volition, since the body is not represented as it should be, or in a state of pristine health: the limb is often experienced crushed; mangled, with fragments of shrapnel in it; or burned, in the state that led to its removal. A phantom limb is something else, not described in textbooks of neurology. It is a deep, vital experience that we do not understand, any more than we understand pain. It is like a movement of the soul, a trepidation so powerful that it pries open the hermetic doors of time and rescues a frozen segment of life that is neither past nor present; a magic act of the body so portentous that it resuscitates a dead and decomposing limb, or reconstitutes it from burnt ashes, guides it across the gulf of time, and reimplants it on the parent trunk, in order to defy catastrophic adversity with the simple affirmation that says, "I am alive."

Pain Willed

Our professed cultural orientation regards pain as eminently undesirable. It is something to be avoided, or opposed. Pain is the enemy, to be fought against with unremitting pugnacity, and deserving neither respite nor mercy. This is why we are much bewildered when we see human beings forswearing their natural allegiance and seeking to embrace pain. It is as if we witnessed treason most foul against the species, a crime more unreasonable than any which may be imagined. And yet pain is sometimes actively pursued, whether it be to brave it, to confront it, or to test it, and thus be tested by it. The pain-seeker may wish to better see himself in the foe's cool eyes, as a lover seeks his own image, his own body, through the eyes and body of the beloved. The ostensible motives are always grandiose: a test of human powers, a means to transcend the human condition, or an offering to supra-individual agencies, kin, country, or the deity.

In the industrialized world, the occasions have become rare in which public display of outright self-inflicted torture takes place unforestalled. The spectacle of a pilgrim stripped to the waist and carrying spinous cactuses suspended from his neck, that every step be marked by nettling to his trunk, is now confined to the narratives of anthropologists—and to my child-hood memories of processions at the shrine of Our Lady of Guadalupe. But the universality and perdurability of such prac-tices should warn the complacent. There is a common streak of self-destructive unreason in all of us; its claim to legitimacy may be disregarded only at our own peril.

In a place on our planet many thousands of miles east of the central dome of Our Lady of Guadalupe, a group of young Chinese novices ready themselves to become Buddhist monks. Part of the ceremony has already taken place during the preceding ten days. The evening before the third and last part of the ceremony, or *p'u-sa jieh*, the barber has been very busy shaving clean the scalps of all male and female candidates. Lay brothers have also submitted to the shearing, while the lay sisters have only a small square shaved on the top of the head. There is much merriment in this garrulous group of young novices, although it is a hushed-down, restrained kind of merriment, as befits those who have chosen a life of spiritual pursuits. The cause of the jesting is the marking of the scalps. The thin, high-cheekboned, hairless youths with shiny pates, clad in loose monkish robes, gather in groups among the older monks and kneel down one by one, taking a string in their mouths. The opposite end of the string is held taut at the back of the neck by another monk. The purpose is to establish a "central axis," as an architect or a draftsman might have done, in order to trace a series of marks on the scalp. Various patterns in rows of circular dots are drawn by means of a hollow reed dipped in ink. If the marked pattern is not deemed correct, the monk wipes it off with a piece of cloth and starts all over, until the marks are placed the right way.

Then begins the ceremony. After a solemn ritual in which a red parcel is given to each novice, all congregate in the central court of the temple. Leading monks and attendants surround each novice, who kneels down after wrapping his praying rug tightly around his neck, while holding the red parcel in his hands. This bundle contains twelve to fourteen small black cones about one centimeter high, made from a combustible material

obtained from the decaying bark of a tree—that is, a form of
moxa. The monk standing in front of the kneeling novice smears
a wax made from dried longan pulp on the thumb of his left
hand. He takes the cones from the little red parcel tendered
him and touches them at the base with his wax. The cones can
now stick to the scalp, where they are deposited at the places
indicated by the rows of circular ink marks. With a lighted
paper, the tips of the cones are set on fire. The monk or his
attendants hold tightly the head of the novice, forcefully pressing
it from both sides, as if to hold it in a vise. This way, it is
immobilized completely. If, on account of the pain, the head
should jerk, the cones would be displaced, or toppled, and the
scars produced would form the wrong pattern.

All the while the novice and the attendants have been con-
tinuously reciting a prayer to Sākyamuni (one of the epithets
applied to Buddha):

Nán   wú   běn   shīh   shíh   jiā   moú   ní   fú

南　無　本　師　釋　迦　牟　尼　佛

("I take my refuge in thee, thou original master Sākyamuni.")
The twelve or so glowing points draw nearer and nearer the
scalp; and with the progress of the flame, the tempo of the
prayer rises equally with its pitch. Quicker and quicker, and
higher and higher: the degree of anxiety may be read in the
cadence and tone, as if on the dial of an electronic instrument.
At last the fire reaches the skin, and a cry of pain emerges from
the throat. The burning flame still lives unextinguished, on
account of the wax, for approximately one minute, long enough
to leave a permanent, visible scar. A Danish observer recorded

seeing people who stood the ordeal without flinching, but also "old men and boys throwing their arms around the knees of the leader, as if they were all of the same juvenile years. While this occurred among the men, I did not see a single nun or lay sister who did not take the branding, whether of three or twelve marks, without a sound or quiver."[4]

Practical people that they are, the Chinese never felt comfortable with these carryings-on in their midst. A memorial to the emperor dated A.D. 819 refers to people who "scorch the crown of their head and burn their fingers." If the emperor does nothing to stop this, warns the official report, "then for certain they shall cut off their arms and slash their bodies by way of sacrifice." Prophetic words. The reverend monk who inscribed the "diplomas" (sacred scrolls) given to the ordained monks at the described ceremony—well into the present century—was noted by the Danish observer to hold his writing brush between the thumb and middle finger. The rest of the fingers of his right hand, and two of his left hand, had been reduced to short stumps by self-inflicted sequential amputations. This elderly holy man could remember the dates at which he had voluntarily cut off his fingers: the fifth right digit on the second year of the Republic; the second right digit on the fifth year of the Republic; the fifth left digit on the sixth year of the Republic; and so on. The characters that he lovingly inscribed on his scrolls, spelling Buddhist prayers, had a beautiful red-purplish hue. The ink he used in these tracings was prepared from a thick paste that incorporated blood as an ingredient—blood from the profuse hemorrhages that had attended each of the self-inflicted finger amputations.

Evidently, voluntary suffering undertaken "to honor Buddha"

or to promote the development of inner life can adopt many forms, from shutting oneself up in a cave, like the Western saints, to willfully ascending—or descending into—the funeral pyre. The West counts many examples in which the attempts to suppress this behavior generated madness more dreadful than the madness they were meant to suppress. But the supremely practical Chinese came to grips with the dark impetus of self-destructiveness. By 1649, an imperial decree had forbidden the ceremony of branding until after the delivery of "diplomas" to the newly ordained monks and nuns. The reason was that a fee had to be paid to the state for each "diploma" extended. If the monk or nun had already obtained the visible scarification marks that proved his or her ordination, the likelihood was high that the fee would go unpaid: money matters, of course, ought not to trouble the spiritual.

In the few decades since the Buddhist ceremony of ordination was described by a Western traveler, violent jolts, profound changes have taken place in Chinese society. But I would be skeptical of official pronouncements telling us that the contemplative were all turned into internationalist fighters, and that the mystical became forward-looking builders of the New Order. Ten to one, if history teaches anything, the roads of China are still trodden by people with fewer fingers and toes than is normal for our species, and this through no accident or congenital mishap. What no doubt changed is the manner of dating the loss: a finger gone the first year of the Cultural Revolution, or a toe vanished in coincidence with the arraignment of the Gang of Four.

It would be idle to attempt a worldwide survey of self-inflicted violence. But a particular form of it, affecting multitudes and striking in waves, like epidemics, merits at least a passing glance. Tertullian mentions the festival called Dies Flagellationis, at which youths flogged themselves before the altar of Diana, while Herodotus (*Euterpe*, Book II, Ch. 41) speaks of like folly in Egyptian worshipers and priests. Saint Augustine denounced the whole lot of pagan practices but praised a pagan, Seneca, for being more outspoken than any of his contemporaries in his condemnation of the dreadful rituals. It is easy to recognize the Iberian philosopher's authorship in the sinewy paragraph quoted by Saint Augustine:

> One man cuts off his male organs; another gashes his arms. If this is the way they earn the favor of the gods, what will they do when they fear their anger? The gods do not deserve any kind of worship, if this is the kind of worship they desire. . . . Men have been gelded to serve a monarch's lustful pleasure; but no tyrant has ever ordered a man to castrate himself with his own hands. . . . They gash themselves at the temples; they offer their blood as sacrifice. If anyone had time to notice what those people do, and what they have done to themselves, he would discover things so unbecoming to men of honor, so unworthy of free men, so incongruous for men of sane mind, that he would have no hesitation to call them mad, if they were not so many sharing the same frenzy. As it is, their title to sanity rests on the number of the insane. (*City of God*, Book VI, Ch. 10)

The collective frenzy went on and off, ever resurging unabated, for centuries. In the West it took a corporate mien with the institution of the Brotherhood of Flagellants, traced by scholars to fourteenth-century Hungary but quickly spreading to the rest of Europe. Remnants of this sect, allowing for inevitable differences due to time and cultural setting, are still to be found in our day in the Southwest of the United States, where Los Hermanos Penitentes now and then horrify the public, mobilize the police, and shock a middle class that prefers to systematically ignore the shady recesses of the human mind. In its beginnings, the Brotherhood compelled the adherence of thousands. Clad in somber sackcloth, singing hymns, often preceded by "persons of consequence" attired in rich robes and carrying banners and tapers, their processions through the cities hardly lacked panache. They found an illustrious biographer in the Abbé Boileau, whose Latin work *Historia Flagellantium: de Recto et Perverso usu Flagrorum apud Christianos* (Paris, 1700) sets the record straight in all that pertains to the correct use of the "discipline of the scourge," as it was then called, besides constituting an authoritative historical source on the excesses of the barbarous custom.

Well into the seventeenth century, Colmenar, a French traveler, described the public procession of Holy Friday at Madrid in a book originally entitled, not without irony, *The Delights of Spain and Portugal*. French travelers writing on Spain have not earned universal plaudits for equanimity; decidedly less so at that time, at the nadir of Franco-Hispanic coexistence and at the zenith of their political rivalries. Colmenar's narrative is nonetheless instructive, especially a paragraph that illustrates the curious turn that self-mortification had then taken:

There are some who take this exercise [of the discipline] from a true motive of piety, but there are others who practice it only to please their mistresses, and the gallantry of it is of a new kind, one unknown to other nations. The good Disciplinarians wear gloves, and white shoes, a shirt of which the sleeves are tied with ribbons, and they have a ribbon attached to their cap, or to their scourge, of the color which most pleases their mistresses. They scourge themselves by rule and on a fixed and settled plan, with a whip of cords that terminate in a little ball of wax with pieces of pointed glass stuck in it. He who flogs himself with most vigor and address is considered the most courageous. When they come across a good-looking woman, they take to scourging themselves so deftly that their blood rains even on her, which is an honor that the belle never fails to acknowledge to the gallant Disciplinarian. And when they find themselves in front of the house of their mistress, then it is that they redouble the blows with greater fury, tearing their backs and shoulders. The lady, who sees them from her balcony, and who knows the real intention, is grateful in her heart, and will not fail to take it all into account.[5]

The narrative is complemented by descriptions of all manner of flesh mortification styled in the processions: carrying crosses of enormous weight, and swords and knives so placed against the body that movements produce lacerations of the skin, deep into the muscles. The penitents walk masked, followed by masked servants who assist them and support them in their dreadful progress.

Barbarous times. Inhumane practices. Abhorrent customs. We must congratulate ourselves for our luck, which spared us from being born in times so unenlightened. But this being so, I cannot explain why the reading of the ancient narratives should call forth images of contemporary life. The face of the flagellant, disfigured by mortification, becomes the scarred visage of a football player recently interviewed on television, a man who was crippled by multiple traumas sustained during his life as an athlete in professional football. Asked if he could say why he underwent such tortures, the former athlete replied by asking the reporter whether she loved her husband. And upon her saying, "Yes, of course," he replied, "Well, I love football. Now you can understand." Surely, no common elements exist between a man disabled by misunderstood piety and a man lamed by the intimate persuasion that love of football and love of husband are qualitatively and quantitatively indistinguishable. Colmenar's narrative of the Portuguese Holy Week processions describes a crowd exhorting the penitents to a higher pitch of self-inflicted cruelty, and heaping abuse upon the timid, who restrain the strength of the lashes out of cowardice or lack of zeal. But I do not know what the Portuguese crowd looked like. Perhaps this is why I picture in my mind the crowd of today's boxing arena. And instead of penitents, I see the thousands—tens of thousands?—of young men of this country, who yearly sustain serious injuries, and continue to play the game with torn ligaments and pulled muscles, oblivious to pain on account of the roaring of the crowd, and the conviction that something greater than bodily pain is at stake through their stoicism; something so grand that by its side the integrity of bones and flesh is as nothing; so majestic as to make fractures and internal bleeding seem trivial accidents.

It is patently absurd, of course, to draw any comparison. The flagellant of yore intended to hurt himself, whereas athletes and daredevils today incur injuries *apparently* unintended. However, if I were pressed to find one respect in which the two coincide, I believe I could produce it. It is that both ancient and modern "self-disciplinarian" must have searched, among the crowd of pitiless onlookers, for a pair of cherished eyes shining with tender compassion. And upon encountering their glance, both must have hoped that their seemingly senseless sacrifice might somehow "be taken into account."

What the Touch Feels

You have to see the charming Italian churches of the Renaissance, with their façades strikingly painted in stripes, in order to understand how it happened that during his daily activities master Benedetto Castelli (1577–1643), one of the oldest disciples of Galileo, should come across a large number of bricks painted on the same surface half black and half white. Like all educated men of his time, he was interested in architecture. Castelli was Italian and grew up in the sixteenth century, which is a way of saying that his mind was keen and trenchant, his temperament livelier than the standard in other latitudes, and his intellect very much in contact with the life of the senses. All this explains why he would notice that bricks so painted, after lying in the sun for about one hour or a little more, were perceptibly warmer on the part painted black than on the part painted white. No doubt his personality, as described, also determined that he should abstain from endlessly ruminating on his observation, and decide to communicate his finding in a jesting and scathing fashion to his peers.

Conspiracy came naturally to those men. Castelli did not prepare a learned monograph for the Academy. Rather, he was of a mind to make his finding into a tool to deflate the egos of the haughty gentlemen who sat listening to learned briefs at the Academy. To this end, he enlisted as confederate a young pupil of Father Confalieri, celebrated philosopher at the Gregorian College, and the two of them confabulated to ask the famous scholar for an explanation of the observed phenomenon. With this twist, however: they would present the priest the *reverse* of the result; that is, they would say to him that the bricks had become heated more on the white part than on the black.

Imagine the scene. The two searchers after true knowledge are received at the college by the most exalted guru with due pomp and circumstance. They manifest their admiration for the depository of the wisdom of the ages, humbly apologize for coming to him with trivial questions that take him away from his momentous researches, and then ask him for an explanation of the temperature differential in the bricks—winking at each other when he is not looking.

The sage clears his throat, adopts a solemn pose while making sure that he still has a sizable audience of students around him, and embarks on a grave disquisition on the nature of colors and temperatures. He speaks of essences and ethereal principles; of arguments advanced by the ancients and confuted by the moderns; of bubbles in the conformation of matter, which are more numerous in white than in black substances; of formal whiteness, nominal whiteness, apparent blackness, real blackness, and so many other subtle philosophical matters that the questioners begin to think the joke is on them. The truth of it is that Father

Confalieri displays so subtle and long-drawn a philosophy to prove the wrong fact that the conspirators think they have already paid in excess for their ill intention. However, the joke has to be carried to its end. After the long peroration is finished, the inquirers fake embarrassment: they have confused the terms of the question; what they really meant was the reverse of what they had stated. The philosopher, of course, is not about to admit that his long reasoning was mistaken. He sticks to his conclusions. So they all decide to meet the next morning in order to confirm or refute, by the then all-pervasive method of experimental observation, the conclusions arrived at by unassisted reasoning.

At the appointed hour they gather at the construction site. The old scholar carefully feels with his hand the black and the white halves of the selected bricks, amidst the expectation of the students; and—who would have expected differently?— does not believe the data of the senses. Oh, the power of philosophical conviction! If the facts disagree with a cherished hypothesis, is it not automatic to blame the facts for inconsistency? Unfortunately for our scholar, this is the Renaissance: not everyone shares his heroic reverence for the syllogism. The students are divided. There are heated exchanges in which speculative purity weakens by degrees at the rude puissance of experiment. The metaphysicians put up a gallant resistance, however. They cry foul, insist that there are shading artifacts, demand that the experiment be repeated under different conditions, and with bricks made of different materials. The experimentalist group rejoins that the original question referred to *this* brick only, but grants repetition of the experiment for the next day.

The comings and goings of this coterie of robed scholars and students must have astounded the masons and bricklayers who watched the proceedings, mouth open, from the scaffolds. At last truth prevails. Black *is* warmer. The speculative thinkers yield, but their leader takes his revenge by foisting upon his listeners a new long-winded dissertation. This time the most exquisite argumentation and sublime reasoning are summoned to prove exactly the opposite of what he had first concluded.

Castelli may not have learned much from this forced exposure to first principles. As a teacher he did not need it; his superb didactic ability reminds us of nothing less than the Socratic dialogues. Teaching a young pupil, he asks:

"What colors feel warmer to the touch, the dark ones or the light ones?"

The child answers, without thinking: "The dark ones."

"Tell me, where is there more heat, in the sun or in the shade?"

"In the sun."

"But dark colors resemble the shade more than the light ones. So, tell me again, what color is warmer, black or white?"

"White."

"Think a little. From which object comes more light to your eyes, from the black or from the white one?"

"From the white one."

"Now look at this brick, one half painted white, the other half black. Listen to what I tell you. If we were to shoot twenty-five pistol shots with red-hot balls into the white part of the brick and twenty-five into the black part; and of those shot into the white part twenty were to bounce back, but of those shot into the black part only five were to bounce back, in which of the two parts would there be more red-hot balls?"[6]

The student seizes the concept: the sun rays are the pistol shots; and since dark objects retain more of them while light objects bounce them back, it is natural that dark objects feel warmer to the touch. By the eighteenth century, the concept of heat absorption could be formulated with elegant precision. Benjamin Franklin, who was not second to Castelli in lucid exposition, set forth his observations this way:

> Try to fire Paper with a Burning Glass. If it is White, you will not easily burn it, but if you bring the Focus to a Black spot, or upon letters, written or printed, the paper will be immediately on fire under the letters.
>
> Thus Fullers and Dyers find black Clothes, of equal thickness with white ones and hung out equally wet, dry in the Sun much sooner than the white, being more readily heated by the Sun Rays. It is the same before a Fire, the heat of which sooner penetrates black Stockings than white ones, and so is apt sooner to burn a Man's Shins. Also Beer much sooner warms in a black mug set before the fire than in a white one, or in a bright Silver Tankard. . . .[7]

Benjamin Franklin actually performed the experiments that Castelli's opponents had demanded. He cut small bits of cloth, paper, cardboard, leather, and other materials into small squares of different colors. On a sunny winter morning he carefully deposited them on top of the snow. When, after some time, he came back to see what had happened, he discovered that the black squares had sunk deep into the snow, whereas the white ones rested on its surface. The materials of colors intermediate between black and white had sunk to intermediate depths, according to their ability to absorb heat from the sun rays.

Some colors, then, absorb and retain heat better than others. But color and temperature remain different things; to speak of "cool" or "warm" colors is, strictly speaking, nonsensical— unless it be poetical, i.e., a form of nonsense generally considered pardonable. Right-thinking people know that colors are picked up by the eye, and temperatures by the touch; and the two sensations are different and independent from each other. Such is the concept of sense perception, grounded upon scientific evidence too voluminous to recapitulate. However, perception is never simple, and there may be cause to question the obvious.

Obviously, to see is not to hear, but there seem to be visual ways of hearing. The experience of listening to music varies according to whether one's eyes are open or closed. When we close our eyes in the concert hall, the music sounds different, not just because we concentrate better by eliminating distracting sights, but because the music now diffuses, as it were, into an ambiance without seats, balconies, or columns. Likewise, when the color red is perceived, it is not *simply* a matter of visual perception. A whole bodily attitude results therefrom: the muscles of the neck and back are tensed, and a mental atmosphere is generated that is congruous with the perception of red. Exactly the same concomitants are never repeated when the perception is of blue, white, or another color—hence the advice to prepare visual aids of a background color that is "restful" to the audience. We do not see red first, then adopt a certain bodily attitude: the reaction is immediate, and we are not aware of it. But psychologists know that motor performance is influenced by the color of the room in which motor skills are tested. Production managers know it, too, since they would never allow delicate manual work to be performed inside rooms painted "hot" red, or "screeching" yellow. Is it correct to say that there is a motor side of vision? Or else the sensation of temperature may be different depending on the color of the enclosure in which the temperature is felt. But if we were subjected to the appropriate test, we would not be aware of three autonomous sensations—color, temperature, muscle re-action; rather, we would say that we feel coolness *in* the blue, or warmth *in* the red, and that we are made tense *by* the particular color. Could it be that the senses overlap, and that colors are apprehended by sight as well as by touch, or that the eyes have a way of seizing sound, albeit different from the ears'?

Here is an idea that is naturally repugnant to the Western mind. Our orientation is analytic, and thus favorable to the scheme that cleaves the senses asunder. Wrote Lucretius, "To each apart/Has been assigned its function, and to each its pow-ers" (*De Rerum Natura*, Book IV, 490). To deny this would be to deny centuries of scientific effort. The eyes are separate from the ears. Our organs of perception are separate windows, each fronting a different segment of the perceptual horizon. Anatomy and physiology have painstakingly demonstrated the autonomy of the nervous system structures serving each of the senses. To suggest otherwise is unthinkable. Lucretius, too, seemed scan-dalized at the mere suggestion (Book IV, 487–89):

Can hearing rectify sight, or touch hearing?
Or else shall taste show touch its mistakes? Is smell
Going to confuse them, or is it sight who will triumph?

And yet, much in spite of all this, the perceptual synthesis takes place somehow. This is undeniable. Non-Western cultures long knew it, and their synthetic conception, though clad in mummeries and irrationality, was not wholly erroneous.

Sooner or later the educated whites in the West had to stop thinking of the existential perspectives and cultural universe of peoples of non-Western tradition as immature or inferior degrees of civilization. And the transmitters of these cultures taught that there is more to seeing, tasting, hearing, touching, and smelling than is understood by these sensations in the scientific-rationalist scheme. The wus of China, the shamans of Asia, the fakirs or dervishes of India and Persia, the bazirs and balians among the aborigines of Borneo, and so many others taught by personal example that sense perceptions are wondrous life states in which stimuli are seized simultaneously by different senses. Their teaching was deeper, since they showed that the senses may be transcended. The senses influence one another; and it is possible to ascend, through sense perception, to levels of consciousness that surpass ordinary experience.

The shaman "feels" the sacred music in his skin. The Huicholes of Mexico, like other Indian groups of the American continent that ritually consume hallucinogenic plants, know that sounds are not for the ear only: colored blotches are created by the drum sounds in their nocturnal rituals. The perceptual synthesis, though a normal occurrence, is enhanced by the consumption of peyote. But whether by natural or artificial means,

levels of consciousness are soon reached that we deem exceptional. The shaman, wu, or fakir evinces a drowsy stare, shiv-
ering, yawning, rolling from side to side. The priest is now
possessed: touch, odor, sound, color, acquire for him a different
meaning. Most spectacularly, he is immune to pain. In the
propitiatory processions of rural China, to describe one example
among many, the wu walks naked to the waist, his hair flowing
loose and disheveled. Long daggers are implanted deep into his
cheeks, so that the blood drips down. Or else a thick needle is
thrust through his tongue, and the bloody spittle drops on sheets
of paper for which the crowd scrambles eagerly: bits of the
paper, imbibed with the devil-repulsing might of the medium,
will make powerful charms to hang over doors, lintels, and beds,
or to fasten tightly to the body of the believers.

I believe that the autonomy of the senses would not be so
dear a concept to us if our scheme of perception had been
derived from Huichole sources. But Huicholes are not neuro-
physiologists. Peyote is to them a sacrament, not a botanical
specimen belonging to a system thick with species, classes, and
genera. Consequently, our theoretical scheme of sense perception was entirely built by somewhat jejune whites, skeptical in
outlook, rational, distrustful of the senses, and systematically
suspicious of any experience that could not be reduced to words
and abstractions. Which is why we have been living by a
watered-down idea of the life of the senses: a scientific-rational
formula that cannot recognize the intercommunicating nature
of perceptions, and which cannot help us in understanding what
it may be to really apprehend, directly and unconditionally, the
objective world by means of the senses.

I suppose my bias is clear: the ultimate understanding of sense perception will require a *redefinition* of perception. It is as much a philosophical problem as it is a scientific one. Whether I am right or wrong it is impossible to tell, but I take heart in the statements made by acknowledged intellectual leaders of our time. Peyote eating acquired some respectability with Aldous Huxley's colorful *J'accuse*: "We cover our anterior nakedness with some philosophy—Christian, Marxian, Freudo-Physicalist —but abaft we remain uncovered, and at the mercy of the winds of circumstance. The poor Indian, on the other hand, has had the wit to protect his rear by supplementing the fig-leaf of a theology with the breech-clout of transcendental experience." Huxley was too astute to believe that a chemically induced trance could be made the ultimate goal of human life. Pharmacology, he knew, will not hand us the Perfect Nirvana. What, then, did he expect from the use of drugs? All he was suggesting was, in his words, "that the mescaline experience is what Catholic theologians call 'a gratuitous grace,' not necessary to salvation, but potentially helpful and to be accepted thankfully, if made available."[8]

Merleau-Ponty, leading exponent of phenomenology in France and foremost critic of the scientific-empiricist scheme of the senses, also spoke for the need to find new formulas that leave room for the transcendental nature of the senses. After a difficult passage in which he discusses the interaction that takes place between percept and percipient, he states:

> . . . I lend my ear, or I look out expecting a sensation, and suddenly the sensible seizes my ear or my glance. I surrender a part of my body to this way of vibrating and of filling the space which is the blue, or the red. As the

Eucharist not only symbolizes an operation of the divine
Grace under a sensible form, but *is* the real presence of
God, makes it reside in a fragment of space, and com-
municates it to those who eat the consecrated bread if
they are inwardly prepared, just so the sensible not only
has a motor and a vital significance, but is actually a certain
way of existing in the world that confronts us from a
given point in space, which our body seizes and assumes
[for itself] if it can; and sensation is literally a communion.[9]

I confess that paragraphs such as this leave me breathless. I
don't know what to say. All that occurs to me is: What! Eucharist? Merleau-Ponty's communion? Huxley's "gratuitous
grace"? When such words are in the mouth of contemporary
Western intellectuals, the "Huichole Textbook of Neurophys-
iology" must not be far behind . . .

HEARING

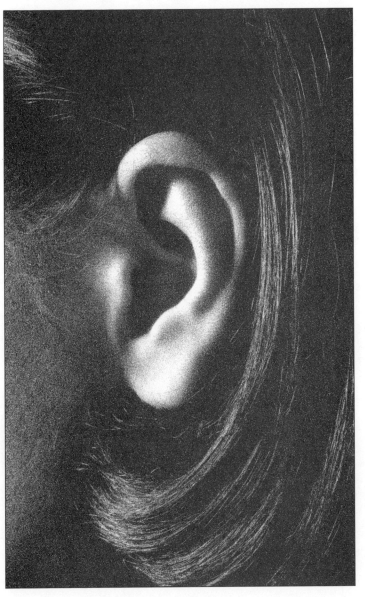

THE ASCETICS of all ages condemned the pleasures of the senses. Excessive indulgence, they remonstrated, makes the sinner resemble a beast. Aristotle, however, allowed two exceptions: the pleasures of vision and of hearing, whose enjoyment, even immoderate, does not debase the human condition. His argument (*Hist. Anim.*, 611b, 26) is as follows. Voluptuous sensations annexed to taste, touch, and smell are shared with all animals. The enjoyments provided by these special senses find their initiation, growth, and culmination in the body. The vices that originate in these pleasurable sensations make man resemble the animals, since animals give themselves freely to the same excesses. It is otherwise with vision and hearing, whose enjoyment comes to full fruition in man only, and is linked to the human mind's capacity to enjoy. The Stagirite's contention is that no animal, except man, is moved by the sight of a beautiful painting, or a landscape, or stirred by deftly combined, harmonious sounds. Excess in the gratification of these senses, therefore, cannot return man to animality. It is exactly the opposite: the more indulgence is permitted in these perceptions, the greater the distance between human beings who partake of those pleasures and the lowly beasts.

Around this hierarchical organization of the senses and their vices an ancient controversy arose. Not everyone agreed on the validity of Aristotle's argument. Those who did, however, never failed to extol hearing as one of the noblest of our faculties, since even in "vice," or excess, it helps to confirm our preeminence among all animal species. They pointed out that the pleasures of other senses are indulged in stealth and in solitude, as if their cultivators wished to hide within four walls an act that they suspected of being a return to animality. In contrast, the enjoyment of music, the highest pleasure of hearing, takes place in the open (Greek amphitheaters were built open to the light of day), and in company. For it is to be remarked, in defense of hearing, that the intention of those who assemble to listen to concerts and virtuoso soloists is not to participate in some communal debauchery but to share the specific delights afforded by sounds in an atmosphere of civilized fellowship and ennobling association.

Verily, this rhetorical defense would be impossible in North America today. In 1986, the press reported mayhem in the wake of popular concerts. About 14,500 fans of the "rap" group Run-D.M.C. congregated in the Long Beach Arena, near Los Angeles, to enjoy their favorite harmonies (if such be the word), but nearly three hundred of their number were induced to mid-summer madness manifesting as violent aggression. In the melee that resulted, forty-five members of the audience were wounded, including a man injured by stabbing. The riot was the fourth in the musical tour of Run-D.M.C. that summer. Performances in Pittsburgh, St. Louis, and New York City had left a bloody total of thirty-nine persons wounded, maimed, or disfigured. It appears that the least placid elements of the listeners' person-alities are stirred by quick and critical perception of "heavy metal," "punk," "rap," and other varieties of maliciously as-sembled sound combinations.

This orgiastic effect of music, studied today with the urgency required by an alarming threat, has been known since the be-ginnings of recorded history. The ancient Greeks were well aware that men are apt to make fools of themselves clapping and leaping, and then induced by degrees into more pernicious and unbecoming forms of conduct under the spell of music. Thus the objection could be made to Aristotle, even by his own contemporaries, that audition-generated excess does not always lead to enhancement of man's differentiation from allegedly lower zoological forms. But rebuttal of the Aristotelian thesis was also attempted on different grounds. The assumption that only man is sensible to the pleasures of sound was, and still is, a matter of debate. Then, as now, many granted to animals the ability to experience similar delights. Aristotle himself was not impervious to conceding that musical appreciation is fairly well diffused in the animal kingdom. He seems to have endorsed the quaint notion that horned owls could be captured by performing dances. Pervaded by the rhythm and melody of reeds and tambourines, and enchanted by the movements of the dancers, the horned owls let themselves go into an imitation of the dancers' steps, "shaking their shoulders this way and that"; and while they were so entranced, catchers sprang behind them, surprising the unwary—but rhythmic—birds.

The power of music over the human mind cannot be overestimated. The story has been told many times, and passes for truth, that Philip V of Spain was "cured" of a depression by the melodious arias of an opera singer hired expressly for the purpose. It is a historical fact that Farinelli (1705–1782), whose true name was Carlo Broschi (he changed it in honor of his benefactors, the brothers Farina), a *castrato* and one of the most celebrated voices in Europe, was summoned by physicians at the Court of Spain out of despair at the brooding melancholy of their master. An age poor in therapeutic resources must have been especially sensitive to empirical observations and anecdotal reports that vouched the mood-altering efficacy of music. This belief was rooted in ancient narratives of the miraculous effects of music: Homer recounting that his warriors' choral singing could stave off the plague; Varro claiming that flute pieces relieved the pains of gout; and, more to the point, the biblical David, on the testimony of Scripture, employing his musical ability to cure Saul's mental derangement by playing the harp.

Surely, the Spanish physicians did not need to refer to any published precedent. It was enough that music everywhere seems to sway men's moods. Solemn strains induce reverence; a lively jig quickens the heartbeat; and piety, like a sediment that is stirred, is set awhirl by the organ's reverberations in the temple. A contemporary of the good doctors had written that the Swiss regiments at the service of the French king were forbidden, under pain of death, to sound the "Ranz des Vaches." For it was thought that under the spell of this music the Swiss mercenaries would be so overcome by nostalgia for their homeland that they were likely to forswear their duty and desert the ranks. It was under these persuasions that Farinelli was recruited by the Spanish royal court.

The singer is lodged near the king's bedchamber. The doctors watch for the right moment. As evening descends and the air grows calm, the order is given: Farinelli intones his sweetest, most touching songs. But nothing happens. The king, unshaved, sullen, distraught, remains sunk in a gloomy dejection behind drawn drapes and closed door. The effort is renewed every evening. Then, after some time, Philip V is suddenly aware of his surroundings. He is attentive, and seems to expect the hour. And when the voice of the artist fills the air in his dark room, it is as if the songs have seeped into the innermost depths of his heart. The servants who arrange the bedroom, and the doctors who come to check the state of the royal patient at bedtime, find him absorbed in the music, while tears well up in his eyes and stream down his cheeks. The next day he opens his door, and shortly thereafter has regained his spirits.

A more skeptical age will adamantly deny Farinelli's curative powers. It will assert that depression is self-limited, and that once the disease runs its natural course, it may regress on its own. But, at the time, the singer receives full credit. His merit is deemed real; not the happy coincidence of finding himself in the right place at the right time, but a God-given "gift," the stuff out of which true miracles are wrought. The king and his entourage manifest their gratitude with largesse. During ten years, Farinelli must intone the same four songs every night for a king who finds no repose without his music. This nightly routine is well paid: the singer is given an influential position at court, earned entirely through his vocal purity, but freely exerted on the political scene.

Good Farinelli! More fortunate than the many who before him wrung power from political dexterity, his life flowed in courtly ease for over twenty years. And when his royal patient and protector died, and discord and enmity loomed menacingly on account of political differences with the successor, Carlos III, the singer had the gumption to pack up his things, bid adieu to the austere halls of Madrid, and head for his native Italy, where he ended his days.

Musical or not, sound wends its way into the very core of our being. The proof is that traces of it remain hooked, like ragged tatters, in the soul's inward recesses. This is why, unexpectedly, we may hear sounds that no one perceives, or words uttered by no one. To "hear voices" is an ominous sign; it is well known in schizophrenia. Yet I will confess to having experienced this astonishing phenomenon. It happened exactly three weeks after my grandmother's burial. The sounds were complex: first the raking sound of the broom that she had used daily for many years, early in the morning; then the creaking of the door, followed by her incongruously juvenile voice admonishing, "*Muchacho*, it is not good to sleep so late."

There is one particular moment at which you are most apt to receive the impression. It is a singular instant, when recollecting yourself from slumber you begin to feel the throb of wakefulness through your limbs. However, sleep has not quite left you; and the precarious forms that haunt the mind in dreams are still by your bedside. It is a segment of life in which time does not exist; it knows neither past, nor present, nor future. Nathaniel Hawthorne gave it a name: the *intermediate space*, "a spot where Father Time, when he thinks nobody is watching him, sits down by the wayside to take breath." Here the ethereal sounds and voices are best heard. Nero, it is said, as he lay half-awake heard the sound of trumpets and groans over the tomb of his mother. Saint Augustine perceived a voice that said, *"Tolle, lege"* ("Take, read"). He took the Bible by his bed and opened it at random. He read (Romans 13:13): ". . . not in rioting and drunkenness, not in chambering and wantonness. . . ." Whereupon he left the life of dissipation he was leading and adopted the ways of saintliness.[1]

How this comes to pass no one can tell. It is the vulgar opinion that the air is charged with spirits and intelligences that foresee the events that afflict mankind, commiserate over their plight, and wish to avert them from calamity. The rationalist disagrees. Physicians say that to hear voices is simply a misrepresentation of one's own thoughts, but don't explain why thoughts should be perceived as words. Auditory hallucinations may be "unformed," as of whistling, rushing, or repetitive sounds (tinnitus), or "formed," when words and sentences are perceived, or when singing and music are represented. Ethereal spoken words and unuttered sentences are heard in psychosis, delirium tremens, and conditions portending the disintegration of the mind. The fact that I perceived the voice of my grandmother does not gainsay this statement; but Socrates heard a demon, and no saner man ever existed.

Ethereal music, however, may occur in deafness. A seventy-five-year-old man, who had been losing gradually his sense of hearing, distinctly perceives an aria intoned by a soprano, and then a baritone. He thinks the radio is on but cannot trace the source of the music. Yet he hears it distinctly, and even better with his deafer ear. All medical tests are normal, and the doctors declare him sane. Other deaf patients report similar complaints. They are not psychotic, and apart from deafness their health is satisfactory. "Do you think I am crazy?" asks one of these to the examining physician. Before 1975 the English language medical literature contained no mention of this singular phenomenon: the vivid perception of musical sounds—single voice, solo instruments, a chorus, or a whole symphony orchestra—by patients who suffer certain forms of deafness.[2]

By what system of preternatural checks and balances does music arise when all other sounds are quieted? Psychologists speak of "releases," as if inner sounds were perpetually tending to spring upward, but were kept submerged under the watery floor of memory by the avalanche of new stimuli that keep them pushed down. A sustained level of sensory input inhibits the emergence of percepts of memory traces within the brain. But let the sensory stimuli cease, as in deafness, or the attention be flattened, as in depression, and the sound memories will reemerge, like stubborn weeds, into the sunlight of conscious awareness.[3]

Nor are all imaginary sounds equally troubling. A melody may awaken the patient in the morning, and repeat itself throughout the day with maddening insistence, but the sound may also be pleasant. Then the listener hums, dances, or sings along, keeping the tempo. The curious fact is noted that church music, hymns and choirs, is most often perceived.[4] It is as if, by heavenly ordained compensation, some patients were soothed for their loss. The irony of music in deafness reminds me of the uncannily strange timing of Jorge Luis Borges's blindness. A more avid reader or more ardent bibliophile it would have been impossible to find. As Muslims viewed paradise in the shape of a sensuous garden peopled with beautiful houris, so Borges conceived the heavenly abode in the shape of an immense library replete with leather-bound volumes. The pressures of making a living interfered with his inclination to spend long hours perusing quartos, octavos, maps, catalogues, and ency-clopedias. One day he was appointed chief librarian at the National Library of Argentina. He saw himself having at last the unhindered opportunity to delve into an immense repository of books, when—lo and behold!—he was blind without remedy. He stood in the midst of interminable rows of books of all the types, in all the languages, and could not make out even the large letters on the back of the volumes. He then wrote:

Nadie rebaje a lágrima o reproche
Esta declaración de la maestría
De Dios, que con magnífica ironía,
Me dió a la vez los libros y la noche.[5]

Which, freely translated, may be put thus:

Let no one's tears debase or slight
This statement of God's mastery
By which, with magnificent irony,
I was given both, books and night.

What Borges called God's "magnificent irony" appears to operate in the coincidental occurrence of deafness and auditory hallucinations. The phenomenon seems to have the melancholy compensation of the full pantry in times of famine: you lament the monotonous fare, but dread the day when it will be exhausted.

Sounds can also kill. Is this surprising for a vibration that sinks through the ear and into the heart? There are life-promoting sounds that enliven our mood and brighten our life. There are also deadly ones. Murderous sound treacherously enters the organism, and, like the henbane poured into the ear of the king of Denmark in *Hamlet*, "swift as quicksilver it courses/ Through the natural gates and alleys of the body" until it claims the whole body for itself. Dutch physicians, in 1972, were first to report the reality of heart-seizing sound. An adolescent girl, upon being awakened by a thunderclap, fell to the ground unconscious, convulsing, and incontinent of urine. At first, it was thought that she had been frightened by thunder. But the symptoms repeated themselves, every time associated with a sudden loud noise, and every time followed by manifestations clearly more severe than those of simple fright. For four years she was seen by eminent specialists, but the attacks, diagnosed as epilepsy, continued to occur. A sudden noise, like a metallic pan falling to the ground, or loud music suddenly emerging from a record player, awakening the girl from sleep, initiated the distressing symptoms.[6]

In the course of multiple examinations, minor abnormalities were detected in the electrocardiogram. But the usual maneuvers that cardiologists apply in their clinical investigations, such as hyperventilation, strenuous exercise, massage to the carotid arteries, or the "Valsalva maneuver" (forced expiration against a closed glottis after a full inspiration), were without effect. The physicians even attempted to frighten her suddenly, but this unorthodox method failed to reproduce the attacks. At long last, the appropriate means to reproduce the disease were found. It sufficed that the patient be asleep, then abruptly awakened by a strong sound (the clinicians used an alarm clock), for a syncopal attack to appear, with all its severe symptoms.

The syncopes were due to sudden, severe alteration of the heart's rhythmicity (ventricular fibrillation), provoked by sound. Cardiac syncopes are potentially fatal: if the normal cardiac automatism is not promptly reinstated, irreparable damage or death may follow. In technical jargon, it may be said that a strong auditory stimulus initiated in the mentioned patient a series of neurophysiological changes with ultimate effect upon the heart. But in layman's terms, is it not appropriate to say that the heart is connected to the ear, and that the patient studied by the Dutch physicians may have manifested an exaggeration of a normal, subtle interrelationship? Thus when we say that a sound, a melody, or the voice of the beloved "reaches deep into our hearts," we are not just speaking metaphorically. We are expressing the intimate conviction that in perceiving, our whole being vibrates in unison with the stimulus; and that hearing is, like all sense perception, a way of seizing reality with *all* our body, including our bones and viscera.

Small wonder, then, that music is credited with the power to awake the passions. Its place in erotic love is averred as prominent. Flute girls were the indispensable adjunct of hedonism at ancient banquets. Gluttony, like sensuality, received no minor help from the right musical background. Do animals respond in like ways? According to Aelian (*De Natura Anim.*, Book XII, 44, and Book XV, 25), the Mysians thought so, because they composed a tune called "Hippothoros" ("The Stallion's Leap"), which they used to sound on their flutes to mares that were being covered. They believed the ardor of equine love to be enhanced by the bewitching strains of this melody. And since the offspring of passionate embraces was (at least for horses) reputedly more wholesome and stronger than the progeny conceived in moderation and restraint, flute-playing must have been an important practice in the cattle-raising industry of Mysia.

For man, the erotic potential of melody is well known. Centuries of experience have not dimmed it in the least. I was amused by the contrivance of a Russian film director who, in a film melodrama produced a few years ago, *Moscow Does Not Believe in Tears*, juxtaposed all amorous scenes of seduction to the sound track of the Latin American popular tune "Bésame Mucho." It seems that Soviet gentility could not withstand the shock of two or three Latin guitars battering in unison at the gates of feminine modesty. The experiment is yet to be done, but there is reason to believe that the same devastation might be caused by balalaikas tuned to the appropriate romantic key in tropical climes, amid palm trees and fragrant fruits. Plutarch, therefore, was justified in admonishing against complacency toward auditory sinfulness in the mistaken belief that incontinence applies to gluttony, lechery, or other activities but cannot characterize any aspect of the function of hearing. To maintain such a thing, he warned, is simply stupid. It is tantamount to believing that "a pot should be proud that it cannot be picked up by the belly, or the base, when it can be easily carried by the ears."

In *8 ½*, the celebrated film of the Italian director Federico Fellini, a man fantasizes that he has garnered in a private seraglio, of which he is the sultan, all the women that ever attracted him during his life. All of them, from the women with whom he was only superficially acquainted to those who became his mistresses, from those he shyly contemplated when he was a pubescent boy to those he boldly approached as a mature man. In this imaginary private harem live all the women to whom he ever attached an erotic thought, no matter how transient or implausible. A prominent place is reserved for the airline employee who announced the flights at an airport where our man had once changed airplanes. He had not seen her but had been touched by her voice: a soothing, sensual, enveloping, and silky sound that survived in his memory. And this is why, as all the others carry on in the fantastic harem displaying their charms for the sultan's pleasure, she alone gads about clad in the composed uniform of the airline, perpetually announcing arrivals and departures.

Much has been written of the erotic suggestiveness of the human voice. Many are those who report having been captivated by its timbre or tone. I do not refer to the high-flown warbles of trained singers—the ravages of their croons and hums, solmizations and falsettos, are only too well known—but to normal spoken diction. Some confess to having succumbed to a lilt, or given in to an inflection. Professional radio speakers, I happen to know, boast no small number of "groupies." In fact, the erotic value of the human voice has made possible a curious sociological phenomenon, "sex by telephone." At least in the large cities of the United States there has been a proliferation of this unique species of private enterprise, which rewards business know-how with an eager, mostly (but not exclusively) male public of consumers eager to pay by credit card for services aurally delivered. The customer, I suppose, craves to be greeted by a voice much like that of Fellini's flight announcer. By the sheer evocative power of voice and imagination, his every whim may be satisfied. And why not? The barriers that physical presence can impose are nonexistent; of all the senses, only hearing is active, and imagination needs no more. But in practice the operation is all squalor: a lonely man dials a telephone number, prepays his fee with a plastic card symbolic of money, and is given in return a feminine voice symbolic of Woman.

Erotic human behavior has been greatly influenced by the invention of the telephone. Social scientists have not devoted enough research to this very important topic. Artists, generally alert to the pulse of emotion, have not entirely neglected it. In the contemporary one-act opera *La Voix Humaine*, with music by Francis Poulenc and libretto based on Jean Cocteau's stage play of the same name, a telephone figures as the central pivot around which revolves a human drama. I must admit that upon hearing this masterpiece for the first time I was not impressed.

A musical ear is one of my notorious deficiencies. In the matter of chords, harmonies, flats, sharps, majors, and minors, I am as a babe in the woods. Leather eardrums were my bequest, and drawn overly taut or slack; the percussions of divas never rang true. On the other hand, I am sensitive to traditional operas, especially the Italian. Turiddu's bite I feel in my ear; *Traviata*'s sexist plot still moves me; and the old-fashioned knifings of Columbine, Silvio, or Scarpia keep me in as deep a trance as any other series subscriber's.

This rudimentary state of operatic sophistication disbarred me from appreciating the subtle nuances of sentiment conveyed in *La Voix Humaine*. No catchy tunes, no flowing arias: only one singer, a soprano, declaiming rather than singing her tormented feelings into a telephone (at least Gian Carlo Menotti's *The Telephone* has two singers, I thought). And Poulenc's music, designed to accentuate the speaker's forlorn mood, follows the rhythms of Cocteau's prose without regard for the churlish expectations of the unrefined. But as the performance progressed, I became aware that the reasons for my insensitivity were not only musical. The dramatic telephone conversation, of which the public can hear only one participant—the soprano—is interrupted at times: Cocteau introduced the irony of a flawed telephone service that cuts the conversation at the most inopportune moments. This detail was a concession to verismo but had the effect of reminding me of another telephone, another drama, and the vivid recollection distracted me from the action on the stage. It is also true that around the telephone of my remembrance moved motley characters more akin to the cast of traditional Italian operas than to the urbane Parisian lady of *La Voix Humaine*. As one drinks to someone's health, I wish to propose my remembrance in honor of these figures of my childhood. Here's to you, unforgettable beings.

Reminiscence of the Black Telephone

In the small, ramshackle drugstore that my mother owned some forty years ago, there used to be a telephone. This circumstance may sound trivial but was actually quite important. It was the only public telephone for an entire city block in the proletarian neighborhood of Mexico City where I grew up. A shiny, black, elegant apparatus lying on the counter, above the shelves supporting arrays of bottles of Glostora ("*para un peinado que enamora*," "for a hairdo that enamors," said the rhyming advertisement) and rows of containers of Nivea skin cream. The apparatus in question was a desk model, the creature of Swedish designers of the Ericsson Company (the telephone companies had not yet been nationalized), and could have sat admirably well on the desk of the richest tycoon, so sober were its lines, so ponderous and distinguished its carriage and profile. Little wonder that all the tenants of R Street, from house number one to number forty-nine, felt a kind of proud right of co-ownership over the dignified apparatus. I mean usuary's sense of property, the kind that custom everywhere gives birth to, and the established order everywhere fears and repulses. So it was that all gainfully employed users within a half-mile radius affixed at the bottom of their business cards—when by rare chance they had them—underneath the label of their trade the appositely foreign-sounding notation "Ericsson 19–10–69," symbol of their access to this modern convenience which they shared with over forty-nine other households.

As an able-bodied youth whose moral future closely depended on being kept busy and off the streets, I was appointed errand boy in charge of notifying recipients of incoming calls. The telephone would ring, and I would be off to number forty-seven, across the street, or farther afield, to number thirteen, conscious of my role as harbinger of anxiously expected tidings, to announce to Mr. So-and-so that he was wanted on the telephone. Nor was my charge without subtleties of performance, or rewards upon correct execution. I had to learn to anticipate when my presence, or my announcement, was going to be received with good cheer, and when unwelcome. And I had to behave accordingly.

At the threshold of Mr. A., the furniture-maker, good sense dictated a loud announcement, cried at the top of my lungs, for all to hear. Mr. A. laid aside his tools, looked round with pride while removing his apron, and followed me of a leisurely pace to take, as he roundly declared, "another order." With Miss B., the butcher's daughter, prudence advised an altogether different technique. First, to run very fast in the direction of her shop, since minutes counted, literally, in my business. Then, close to my destination, to approach nonchalantly, to pretend that one is a boy who walks down the street idly, or plays and talks with other children, without a specific mission to accomplish. All the while, however, to observe the proceedings inside the butcher shop. And when the stern father was distracted wrapping pork chops, weighing eye-of-the-rounds, or ringing the cash register, to obtrude myself into Miss B.'s (Bertha was her name) visual field, and to announce the call. Not by way of spoken utterances, of course, but aided by mime: the mouth moving as in uttering "te-le-phone" without actually emitting a sound, while the right index finger traced circles in the air, in simulation of dialing. To which Bertha replied with a nod, and a glance of intelligence mingled with gratitude, such as I have rarely seen flashing forth from feminine eyes. How she managed to leave the shop unnoticed was her business: each one has his duty, thought I, and mine had been discharged to perfection.

Most messenger boys would be content with delivering their message. Such is, after all, the defining note of their calling. The true perfectionist, however, cannot reduce his activities to so narrow a compasss, and feels compelled to investigate the contents of the message. For how else would he know the proper manner and disposition of delivery if not by foreknowledge of what is being delivered? It is not to some unhealthy propensity for gossip and eavesdropping but to the most commendable professionalism that I attribute my childhood interest in those telephone conversations. There was no booth, no cubicle, no compartment to segregate the speaker from the customers. The telephone sat atop the front counter, and there was little the user could do to shield the privacy of his communications. With these annoying details, Mr. A. seemed delighted. For his calls were clearly meant to impress upon the world the loudly proclaimed notion that he was much sought after: a successful craftsman, a man to whom solicitations were addressed, a businessman who—his card so stated—"took orders" at Ericsson 19–10–69. And Miss Bertha? Miss Bertha of the glaucous, tearful eyes! Miss Bertha of the disheveled locks streaming down the forehead; of the reddened conjunctivas; of the gaunt features and shadow-rimmed, sunken eyes; of the fidgeting right hand that twisted the telephone wire with crispatory movements, if not cupping around the transmitter to ensure that her whispered pleas, emerging from the depths of her heart, would sink unpolluted into the apparatus, then travel converted into electrical impulses, and then be reconverted into sound at the other end of the wire, there to move the obdurate heart of an unseen lover! May she have forgiven an indelicate and precocious street urchin who watched, intrigued by what he did not know and could not have known, the ravages of passion, and the seething, relentless consumption of unrequited love.

Two were the most remarkable users. Both were assiduous callers, and both were blind. But apart from the terrible tragedy of blindness, they had little in common. Mr. Z. was married, tall, corpulent, and self-assertive, a commanding presence in his dark, reflecting glasses. Mrs. M. was demure, lived alone, and moved unassisted, yet with extraordinary nimbleness; one might have said a seraphic presence gliding, not walking, and propelled, not sustained, by her white cane.

To these two extraordinary personages, Mr. Z. and Mrs. M., I owe my first direct canvassing of the terror of sightlessness, and the conviction that hardly a tragedy exists that the human spirit cannot overmaster, or that a stoic and brash temper, roused to its mettle, cannot laugh into insignificance. For impenitence and raw vitality Mr. Z. was peerless. Until then, my childish and tender imagination could conceive no terror more unendurable than the privation of sight. Mr. Z. seemed, at first, to exemplify yet a more wretched condition: condemned to perpetual darkness, he was utterly dependent on a furious termagant of a wife.

To paint the wretchedness and desolation of those who,

having once seen, lose their sight, may be attempted. In this sorrowful employ the pen of Milton shone with unexampled might. But what genius will describe the hellish torments of unhappy married life? As the best relationship in the world may be that which joins husband and wife in harmony, so the most hateful relationship possible, the most venomous and deadly, is that which develops between spouses living in rancorous dissension. Let others look to the introspective rumination of contemporary "psychological" writers. My favorite description of marital estrangement, and that of which I think when I reminisce about Mr. Z.'s plight, is the forceful earthy account of a Chinese novelist of the Ming dynasty:

> Nothing compares to this torment. Tyrants are brutal and harsh, but their malice will spare you if you remove yourself from the palace. Cruel parents abuse you, and force you to toil digging wells all day long, but at night they set you free. Only in a hateful marriage there is no respite. It is as if you lived with a huge tumor in your neck [in the days before surgery]: If you try to remove it you risk your life; but if you keep it you prolong your suffering. In the daytime you find no shelter, and at night your torture worsens. Civil law does not apply; the precepts of your parents are without effect. Your siblings, your brothers cannot help you. The neighbors can only stand by. You may be yelled at and humiliated: no one can offer you solace. You may be abused or beaten: no one can intercede in your behalf. You may wish to live: your spouse wants your death. But if you choose to die, he or she will make you live. It is like using a dull knife, one that has

not been sharpened for generations, and sawing back-and-forth on your neck. Is this kind of piecemeal suffering not worse than the torments endured by the souls in the eighteenth [lowermost] circle of hell?[7]

Mr. Z. pined for years in quiet desperation under these most dreadful conditions. His head was being sawed off with the unspeakable grating of a dull knife "unsharpened for generations," biting away, day by day, on his chine. Whosoever has suffered the pains of conjugal disharmony will understand. Then all of this changed. In the span of the few years that my tenure as messenger boy lasted, I was witness to a transformation. What I saw was, first, callous abuse daily heaped upon a defenseless blind man; then, a gradual turning of the tables; and, last, the manumission of the defenseless invalid with the hearty endorsement of his own, grown children.

Mr. Z. was an educated man. Notwithstanding his blindness he was a professor at the Escuela Normal Superior, then a teachers' college. Among his predominantly female students there were some who must have felt that maternal solicitude, bloom of the feminine bosom, that strongly moves to pity and stirs the desire to protect. So it was that Mr. Z. was soon seen in the company of a young woman who carried his books and assisted him on his way. And by those well-known steps that connect compassion to the sublunary regions of man-woman relationships, teacher and student progressed into a full-blown, though illicit, amorous affair.

The effects on Mr. Z.'s wife were fulminant. Her screams could be heard a mile around. On the memorable day of her disabusement, she appeared at the drugstore asking for a drink for *susto*, i.e., for one of a number of states of mental agitation that, like sudden fright or violent rage, threaten by their intensity to upset corporal health. Attuned as we were to the quaint folk belief, we obliged; living conditions in our neighborhood required us to have on hand an abundant supply. (Therapists, take note: 10 percent magnesium carbonate in distilled water; mix 3:1 v/v with cherry syrup.) Her hand shook uncontrollably as she emptied the glass. When she gained some composure she declared persuasively, if somewhat indelicately, "That blind son of a bitch is going to be the death of me!"

As for Mr. Z., what subterfuges, what contrivances did he deploy? He answered the telephone never knowing whether an unwelcome listener stood behind. He received coded messages . . . in Braille, perhaps? My recollection is of a tall, imposing, darkly bespectacled, middle-aged man uttering cryptic phrases into a telephone. Sentences that were alternatively fatherly, tender, or suggestive, but never free from ambiguity, and almost always beyond my comprehension. There followed scenes of domestic strife, recriminations, loud complaints in which the uncouth wife blamed "that accursed blind man" for all that afflicted her, from recrudescence of migraine to canescence; and a final showdown. But there was no stopping the redoubtable Mr. Z., who, under the goading of Eros, had paradoxically "seen the light."

Strange to recount, Mr. Z.'s grown children sided with him during his war of independence. I saw him last when, proud, undaunted, and unrepentant, he was shown by his eldest daughter into the taxi that took him away from the neighborhood. She inspected his outfit, rearranged a carnation in his lapel, kissed him on the cheek, took him by the arm, and gently assisted him to board the taxi. Assuredly, the interplay of invidious forces that went on in that household was much too complex for a messenger boy to comprehend. But the unusual alliance of grown children and blind father against a shrewish mother was one of the most bizarre domestic combinations that I can recollect. I thought about this singular group when, many years later, I heard for the first time a ribald French song of the nineteenth century that was recorded by musical historians as an example of working-class folklore. The lyrics describe the jealousy of a woman who suspects her man of engaging in excessively familiar gambols with a young *cabaretière*. She sends the children to spy upon their disloyal father, but the brats make common cause with the unworthy man. In the end, they report their detailed observations to the mother, and end with their own, callously unfilial conclusion:

> *Il a raison, s'écrièrent les enfants.*
> *Il a raison de suivre celle qu'il aime,*
> *Et quand nous serons grands,*
> *Nous ferons tous de même.*

("He's right, exclaimed the children./He's right to trail the one he loves,/And when we grow up/You bet we'll do likewise.")

For all that Mr. Z. exuded earthiness and Rabelaisian effrontery, Mrs. M. was pure ethereal immanence. I never knew where she lived. It was never my duty to announce incoming calls for her at any of the forty-nine dwellings (many with labyrinthine inner subdivisions occupied by multiple families, or *vecindades*) included in the territory that I proudly might have called my jurisdiction. Instead, she would materialize at the drugstore, rarely assisted by a guide, to request permission to use the telephone. She would approach it purposefully, with hardly a groping motion to betray her condition. Her appearance was striking. A woman in her late thirties or early forties, her youthful dress often stood in shocking discrepancy with her years and ripe somatic conformation.

Imagine a girlish, pink-laced dress, all lustrous taffetas at the bodice, and skirt that terminates four finger breadths above the knee. Imagine, next, this childish garment worn by a busty, mature woman of opulent forms, and you have an idea of the garish vulgarity that transpired. The picture, however, is incomplete. To this description must be added the sobering realization that the woman thus clad was blind. It is with this single element of her description that all judgments were instantly suspended. For this woman, to whom it was automatic—at first sight—to ascribe a faulty character, a deranged mind, or at least a lack of esthetic sensibility, was suddenly revealed to the observer as a pitiable victim. Was she misled by envious and perverse counsel, or exploited by some irresponsible dressmaker? Or did she supplant the conventional visual criteria that everyone uses in selecting clothes, and choose her own dresses based exclusively on nonvisual perceptions, the rustling of fabrics, the feel of crossribs, and the palpatory ascertainment of their cut and proportions?

Mrs. M.'s persona was optical illusion incarnate: she appeared under one guise at first sight, and under a different one at a second; vulgarity was seen by rapid examination, and sheer pathos by attentive canvassing. More than one obtuse libertine was attracted by the tawdry vulgarity of her external appearance; more than one was shocked by the spectacle of her blindness. Such a one approached her from behind, anticipating, from her appearance, commerce with some meretricious trollop, only to be thrown into confusion by the sudden confrontation with an eyeless face, a visage in which the orbits had been emptied of their contents, and in which the mutilation was not always veiled by the modesty of sunglasses.

The object of her passion was perfectly congruous with her personality. I heard it from my mother that a professional radio broadcaster held the receiver at the other end of the line during Mrs. M.'s long telephone conversations. Love, it seems, had shot its darts through invisible waves, and had made her a target at God only knows how many kilocycles of frequency. She disappeared from the neighborhood as mysteriously as she had arrived. Whether in disillusion, or to everlasting contentment in erotico-auditory bliss, I do not know. But I feel certain that Plutarch, in his quaint kitchen metaphor, would have written her off among the number of those who, like pots, were "carried about by the ears."

Having grown into manhood many years later, I was to discover the strange fascination that lies in listening to a cherished voice through the telephone in total darkness. The evocative powers are thus summoned best, as if by magical conjuration. And like all true magic, this operation is best performed in the thick of the night; for it is at night that the demiurgical might of a human voice is exerted in full force. I understood then how much more vulnerable the telephone users of my remembrance must have been, who had no visual perceptions to distract them from vocal fascination.

Question three of Book VIII of Plutarch's "Table Talk" (*Questiones Convivales*) is devoted to this very problem: why sounds carry better at night than in the daytime. Voices appear more sonorous at night; not only their volume, but the precise details of the articulation come to us undisturbed. In this, says one of the convivials, a special favor of Providence may be discerned: the accuracy of our hearing is enhanced at a time when our vision is most impaired, as if a divine compensation repaid to our ears for what is taken away from our eyes. But the Greeks' scientific spirit is skeptical; though granting the existence of divine favor, it must explain the proximate physical causes. Hence, the doctrines of Epicurus are invoked, which explain the phenomenon as follows.

Matter is composed of atoms. Air itself consists of atoms dispersed in the great void. During the day, which is warm, the atoms are loosened about and separated. An approaching sound is thus likely to collide with the loose particles, and thereby endures delays and deformities. Heat dilates matter, whereas cold contracts its substance. At night, under the influence of coolness, the atoms of air are compacted together, leaving empty spaces at the sites they formerly occupied. It is natural that a sound should run unimpeded when it courses through a medium that has much emptiness in its structure. If its route is clear, sound travels free; but when it encounters particles along its way, like highway robbers that seize it and detain it, it is smothered. Yet, for all its Epicurean origins, this theory is a weak one. As the dinner guests in Plutarch's "Table Talk" derisively put it, the theory is one with "much emptiness" in its formulation. Like the air it postulates, free passages and vacuums exist everywhere in its substance, through which doubt creeps in.

If the Epicurean hypothesis were true, stormy nights would be more sonorous than clear ones, for the atoms in air are then pushed together in one place, leaving great gaps through which sound may pass. Or else a cold day would be more sonorous than a hot summer night. But neither of these circumstances obtains. Anaxagoras, therefore, advances a new hypothesis: sound is vibration perceived. Is Anaxagoras a visionary, precursor of modern physics? Not quite. His explanation of why days are more sonorous than nights is imaginative, but fantastical as well. He reasoned that this was a consequence of a general background noise existing during the day. The sun moves the particles that exist in air, since we see that when a beam of sunlight falls upon these particles, or motes, they are set motioning in eddies, or quivering. And since their motion must be accompanied by some sound, we have to infer that during the day there must be background hissing that interferes with hearing. At night, however, the motes are still, and their hissing ceases. And this is why nights are quieter than days.

One of the learned convivials introduces a new idea. Aristodemus of Cyprus, a man not known for any other contribution, squarely unfolds before us the notion that our current jargon calls a "psychological threshold." If night seems more sonorous than day, he says, it is not because the air and its particles have ceased churning. It is because we are better disposed to listening. For what rouses us to words and deeds at night is not something insignificant. Night is the time we devote to sleep and repose. We are not likely to upset this routine, unless it be under compulsion from some extraordinary occurrence, or at the prompting of some emotion. And this is why voices travel with greater force, or our ears are keener in receiving them.

Darkness and the human voice: a mysterious synergism believed important enough to deserve the table talk of Plutarch and his dinner guests. Their odd reasonings, their antiquated arguments, reveal the blind persons of my childhood in a new light, though too late to advert to sympathy, or compassion. If I could, I would speak to you, Mr. Z. and Mrs. M.: I understand the immensity of your plight, and I pity you. Both of you were foredoomed; sight alone would not have sufficed to guard you from the spells and conjurations of the human voice. For the baneful combination that felled you is one for which no remedy is known: outward shadows, inner desires, and the malignant allurement of a human voice.

SMELL

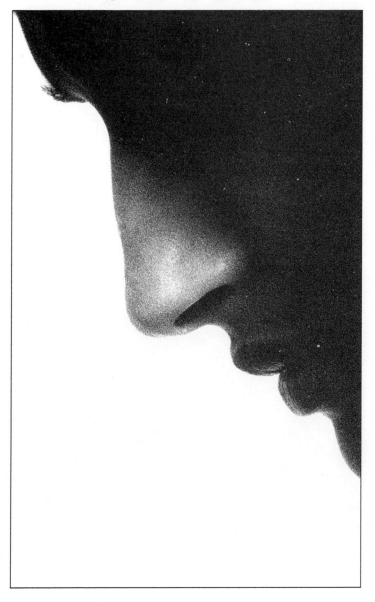

Condillac as Pygmalion

ETIENNE BONNOT DE CONDILLAC (1714–1780) maintained that all human cognition rests upon the perceptions conveyed by the senses. All that we know, all our ideas, he believed traceable to sense perceptions; without these man could not have invented a language or attempted the coarsest speculation. The simplest of inferences, or the most rudimentary calculation, would have been impossible. Conversely, he maintained that a single one of our senses would have made us fit to leave the primeval cave.

To illustrate his thesis, Condillac bids us imagine a statue of peculiar conformation: outwardly made of marble, but inwardly made like the rest of us. Now, to this imaginary statue we shall grant life by degrees (for our life-giving power, being imaginary, is unlimited and may be godlike); and we begin by bestowing upon it the sense of smell. This choice is not random. Olfaction is often deemed the least "intellectual," or the least informative, of our senses: it knows nothing of shapes, numbers, directions, or the material qualities of objects. Nevertheless, Condillac sets out to demonstrate that with this humble and much-maligned tool for all equipment, the human mind is quite capable of lifting itself from the obscure realm of vegetative life to the most splendid and luminous regions of intelligence.

Let us, then, imagine a beautiful Diana, surprised in the strain of the hunt, and suddenly frozen in petrous immobility while tensing her bow. Let her be transported in this frozen state from her sacred woods to a garden, as more fitting to a statue. For she remains, on the whole, a statue. Her flowing robe is fixed in motionless rolls and swells that do not stir with the changing winds, on account of being made of marble, like the rest of her. She cannot hear our footsteps on the gravel path where stands the plinth that supports her. She cannot feel our hand skimming the surface of her sinewy arm. Nor can she see us when we stand squarely in front of her, through her marmoreal eyes without pupils. But since we have just granted her the sense of smell, she perceives the scents of the garden: now the roses of the trellis nearby, now the balsam firs farther off.

If at this time we present her with a carnation, "she will be, with respect to us, a marble statue that smells a carnation; but with respect to herself, she will be the perfume of a carnation."[1] In effect, our motionless Diana is endowed with a single sense that by itself permits no ideas, no judgments on the external world. Bodies, color, texture, extension, and sound are alien to her. Therefore, she cannot conceive her sensations as emanating from something outside herself. She would *be* the smell of carnations, roses, or balsam firs, depending upon what odors the whim of the shifting breezes would waft to her nose. Moreover, each sensation would be perceived as indefinite: she cannot perceive its beginning or its end; for it is only upon reflection on the succession of our ideas that we learn about beginnings and ends. Hence, "with respect to herself" she would *be* a smell of carnations without beginning and without end.

Blissful as this state may seem, it is also transient. For we have made our statue partly human (even though her single claim to this title is our gift, olfaction), and therefore we must expect to have caused the disconsolate state of all things human. She detects a pleasant odor, and experiences something like a joyous dilatation of her being: she has known pleasure. Then a disagreeable, foul stench is brought to her by the garden breeze. This perception will be like an oppressive sufferance, a kind of contraction of her vital horizon: she now has known pain. New sensations bring forth new pains, or new pleasures, and a wider range of potential comparisons becomes available. If she keeps the memory of these two principles—pleasure and pain—she will soon be wishing the one and fearing the other. And how keen her desire to seek the one and flee the other! Having only one faculty, that of smell, our lovely marmoreal Diana concentrates all her emotional sensitivity upon it. Unlike the rest of us, common mortals who must constantly divide our attention among the myriad solicitations of the environment, she focuses all her feelings solely upon odoriferous perceptions. Pleasant aromas she yearns for; unpleasant smells she loathes with equal vehemence.

After some time, the statue that we thought doomed to languish in a dumb, dark, and brutish world of minimal sentience has acquired a mind closely resembling our own. She has attained the knowledge of pain and pleasure, and decided that she prefers the latter. She has called past experience to her consciousness, and realized that there is more than one kind of experience. She has watched the succession of odors, and now anticipates their sequence. With olfaction alone she has constructed memory, discernment, judgment, and abstract notions, such as ideas of number, succession, and duration. With olfaction alone she has acquired what the ancient authors called "passions"—that is, astonishment, hopes, desires, volitions, likes, and dislikes.

There we have our quondam placid statue, now prey to human joys and sorrows. Which shows, as the good abbot of Condillac does not fail to remark, that "with one sense only,

our understanding has as many faculties as with the five together." Further to strengthen this thesis, Condillac proceeds
to consider each of the other senses separately, as he had done
for olfaction. The statue is gradually animated by more human
attributes. And by following what he fancies to be the mental
evolution of a statue thus endowed with one specialized sense
alone, then in combination with one or more of the others, the
philosopher illustrates his conclusion that "the senses teach the
mind."

That Condillac borrowed liberally from the British empiri-
cists, and from John Locke especially, is only too apparent.
Empiricism postulated that when we come to the world our
mind is like a new notebook (*tabula rasa*, "clean slate," was the
expression at the time) upon which the five senses inscribe the
words that will compose all our ideas, even the most abstract.
Needless to say, not all thinkers accepted the empiricist claim
that abstract ideas were born in this fashion; some denounced
this attributed paternity as suspect.

Kant was the boldest. He said that abstract ideas (or, to use
his words, "intellective concepts") are, indeed, born in the mind,
but cannot *derive* from sense perceptions. In the Kantian view,
Condillac's statue may well learn that there are odors, but the
concept of *existence* cannot follow from this learning. She may
know that she perceives, but the concept of *perception* cannot
accrue from the addition of concrete sensible contents, i.e., the
stuff of perceptions. She may learn that fragrant aromas may
be followed sometimes by disagreeable smells, or by other odors,
but the concept of *possibility* can in no way be born of the
experience of perceiving them. In other words, the ideas of
being, possibility, causality, necessity, number, and many others

SMELL   69

refer to relationships that are not sensible, and therefore cannot be "extracted" from sense perceptions by analysis, as one extracts juice from grapes by squeezing them in a press. The relational concepts are not engendered, or abstracted, from sensible phenomena, for one can only abstract what is already present, in one form or another, in the object of analysis.

A venerable philosophical tradition, then, has long maintained that the mind is not, in our beginnings, a virgin notebook. The script of "innate ideas" is already inscribed on its pages. This script is a plan, according to which the mind instructs the senses and commands them to perceive. The mind teaches the senses, instead of learning from them. But if it teaches them, it is because it has knowledge, and this knowledge antedates experience. It is, then, an *a priori* kind of learning, a received set of "innate ideas." Kant, like his antiempiricist predecessors, had no choice but to believe that innate ideas were a gift of the Divine Providence to mankind: a sort of welcome present neatly gift-wrapped and dropped into our skull by the powers that protect us and watch us from celestial heights.

The foes of empiricism today need not resort to mystical explanations. Current scientific theories on the phylogenetic development of the brain throughout evolutionary history are compatible with the claim that people can know something of the world innately, that is, prior to and independent of their own experience. "After all," wrote Max Delbrück (physicist, astronomer, and Nobel prize laureate biologist),[2] "there is no biological reason why such knowledge cannot be passed from generation to generation via the ensemble of genes that determines the structure and function of our brain." Therefore, this distinguished twentieth-century scientist was compelled to aver that the Kantian notion of innate ideas and *a priori* knowledge "is not implausible at all. Rather, Kant's claim [of the innateness of abstract concepts] almost hit the nail on the head. These ideas are indeed *a priori* for the individual, but they did not fall from heaven; they are matters of evolutionary adaptation, designed for survival in the real world."

If we now return to the garden that harbors Condillac's statue, we shall be surprised. We expected to find it smashed to pieces after the furious lapidary barrage of the antiempiricist camp, but the beautiful Diana stands intact, and as graceful as ever. Beauty, not soundness of structure, has saved her. Certain images in philosophy surpass in evocative power those of poetry or epic, and are most lasting. Riddles and enigmas, allegories and paradoxes were contrived by thinkers who wished to illustrate or to enliven their arguments. And after the arguments were dismantled, confuted, and utterly undone, the metaphors survived. Think of Zeno's arrow, shot through the air, and never reaching its target; or Achilles' sempiternal despair at overtaking a tortoise that he cannot outrun. Think of the Cartesian natural world, populated by animals that seem alive but are only mechanical contraptions; or the Berkeleyan universe, whose multifarious objects instantly acquire material existence, or vanish into thin air, according to whether they are thought of by someone or forgotten. In this fantastic world belongs the smelling statue of the abbot of Condillac. She will live the life of undying images in her garden: a life of her own, unmindful of the original purposes of her creator.

The poets never thought of a more beautiful apologue. For Condillac's example transforms us, his readers, into life-giving demiurges who say to themselves, "I shall create a soul to which

I shall give sensations that will also be modifications of its being."
And straightaway we proceed to create with our imagination a
marble statue that thinks, and that experiences its being suc-
cessively as an aroma of jasmines, roses, and violets. Because it
knows nothing of existence, it can have no knowledge of death.
And because, at least at the beginning, it has no notions of
duration, it experiences its being as indefinite in time. We have
then created a being so ethereal that it feels itself as perfume
of flowers for all eternity, and so airy and insubstantial that—
literally—it cannot conceive the idea of matter. Was there ever
a poet who thought of more delicate an image, or more romantic
an allegory?

Moreover, the illustration is uniquely apposite. For olfaction
deals with the airy, the insubstantial, and the formless. Unlike
sight, whose perceptions are so rational that they may be analyzed by the laws of geometry, olfaction rejects geometrical
analysis altogether. Still more, smells often defy localization in
space. Sight has regard to the actualities of space, but olfaction
lives in time, and in time mainly. Of all our senses, this is the
one most closely related to time: to the past, because, better
than the others, it evokes memory; to the future, because, more
effectively than the others, it elicits anticipation and awakens
our deepest yearnings.

Of the Good Odors, and the Odors of the Good

Since it is evocative and deals with the unseen, the unfathomable,
and the imponderable, olfaction naturally came to be associated
with the experience of mystics. Indeed, a keenness of this faculty
passed at one time for the mark of saintliness. Saint Jerome

recounts that an avaricious man, wishing to ingratiate himself with the community of monks in which Saint Hilarion resided, brought with him a bundle of chick-peas which he unloaded on a table. Saint Hilarion immediately cried out that he could not bear the stench: "Don't you notice the horrid stench, the foul odor of avarice in the peas? Give it to the cattle, and see whether the brute beasts can eat it," he said. Presumably, by special divine favor the ability to detect avariciousness by in-halation was made extensive to cattle on that day. For when the holy man's recommendation was followed, the cattle broke their fastenings and ran wildly, bellowing in terror. Jerome insists that Hilarion "was enabled by grace to tell from the odor of bodies and garments, and the things which any one had touched, by what demon or with which vice the individual was distressed."[3]

Saint Pachomius must have shared this gift, at least insofar as the ability to detect feminine sexual misconduct was con-cerned. When the cloak of a possessed girl was brought for him to examine, he discovered that she had a lover. Collin de Plancy, a nineteenth-century French scholar, says in his remarkable *Infernal Dictionary*[4] that a priest from Prague was also blessed with this extraordinary ability by which he could recognize women of loose morals. Plancy adds this uncharitable comment, that "in order to have developed his sense of smell to so high a degree of perfection, it must have been necessary in the course of his ministry to come in very close contact with a great many of them." From various passages of this work, it is clear that the author was disaffected from the Church when the first edition appeared, but reconciled himself with his faith at the time of publication of the second: the gibe disappears in late editions of his dictionary, which is thus considerably dein-fernalized.

Under the entry "Olfaction," Plancy refers to Book XIII of the treatise by Girolamo Cardano (1501–1576), "On Subtility," where it is contended that a good sense of smell betokens spirituality, because the dry and warm nature of the brain tends to render olfaction ever more powerful (a direct connection between nose and brain is among the most enduring myths; up to the eighteenth century it was widely believed that nasal discharge originated from the brain and oozed to the exterior), and those cerebral qualities are also apt to render the imagination more fertile and loftier. The author of the *Infernal Dictionary* correctly denied any connection between olfaction and the moral sense. He was right in doing so. In his own age, in the year 1859, a savant presented before the Silesian Medical College, to the complete satisfaction of that learned body, a peasant who could smell out thieves, track lost objects and human footprints, and identify individual animals from flocks, all by his uncanny (or canine) sense of smell. Nothing in his moral personality was deemed worthy of being recorded for posterity.[5] Likewise, it is said that experienced perfumers are able to distinguish an as-tonishing number of different scents. Now, far be it from me to cast aspersions upon the members of this honest trade: as a group, one cannot say that they are distinctly unholy. But neither is it possible to say that perfumers and cosmetologists have furnished the heavenly legions with a disproportionately large number of the blessed.

Nevertheless, sweet perfumes and celestial bliss would seem naturally joined. Mystics are unanimous in describing other-worldly landscapes as suffused of strong smells, and those in which the just are rewarded as unfailingly sweet-scented. There, to believe Dante, even the Virgin Mary is like a rose; and the Apostles, twelve lilies "whose fragrance led mankind down the good path" (*Paradiso*, Canto XXIII, 73–75). Indeed, the whole of paradise is an Eternal Rose, whose ranks of petals are the souls of the Blest: in a magnificent poetical image, Dante integrates the mystical concept of the immensity and refulgence of that rose with the idea of the praises to God that emanate from it like an inebriating perfume (Canto XXX, 126). For Saint Bernard, the teachings of Christ are comparable to the aroma of flowers in full bloom, since they utterly pervade our lives, and exert their soothing influence from any and all directions. Through the Savior's teachings, said Saint Paul in his Second letter to the Corinthians, we become "the fragrance of Christ for God, alike those who are saved and those who are lost; to these an odor that leads to death, but to those an odor that leads to life" (2:14–16).

Nor can it be supposed that these were purely metaphoric allusions to the saintly life. We who live in a sanitized, de-odorized, and ever more artificial environment often fail to grasp the directness implicit in these ancient sayings. We see metaphor where descriptive realism was intended. The expression "odor of sanctity" is obsolete, but when rarely it is used, and it is said of someone that he "lived in an odor of sanctity," most of us would understand that he lived a life of righteousness and virtue, like a saint. This, however, was not at all what was meant. Originally, the expression meant just what it said, namely, that the saintly were perceptibly odorous—a quality that faithful and unbelievers alike, if sound of nose, could easily confirm. Upon varied testimony we know that Saint Francis of Paul smelled like musk, and that Saint Joseph of Copertino's body exhaled a wonderful aroma that clung to his clothes; Copertino's contemporaries could compare the scent to no known odorant, natural or artificial, but those who perceived it were left in a state of mute delight and admiration. The odor of Saint Cajetan was described more precisely, and its origin more clearly ascertained: his biographer says that Cajetan smelled of the bloom of the orange tree, and that this was so most certainly because he was a virgin (*certissimum profecto ejus virginitatis indicium*).

The odoriferous qualities of the heavenly legions, however, could not be described succinctly. The odor of sanctity is variously consigned in hagiography as musk, lavender, amber, cherry blossom, fern, spices, the aroma of roses, violets (these two flowers most commonly mentioned), lilies, carnations, myrrh, and frankincense. In some cases the aroma could be compared to no known odorant. Moreover, not all the saints came in scented versions, and those who did were not scented all the time. Of the emanations that diffused out of the body of Saint Catherine of Ricci, a hagiographer says that "the Lord permitted some to smell this perfume, but to others He did not allow it, and even those who perceived it once did not perceive it always." The odor of sanctity, then, could be constant or intermittent, and easily identifiable or complex and indescribable.

The holy odor could also be simple or compound. That of Saint Lydwine, for instance, impressed not only the sense of smell but stimulated the taste as well. "It was as if one had eaten ginger, clove, or cinnamon: the strong and spicy flavor softly bit the tongue and the palate," wrote a contemporary. Moreover, the saintly emanations could be perceived during life, or after the mortal body of the saint had perished. In some instances the smell was only apparent years after interment: hagiography tells of more than one exhumation during which the bodily remains were discovered miraculously incorrupt, and the crypt was filled with a sweet perfume, instead of the expected foul stench of organic decomposition.

In the face of so much portent, reason is humbled. Leave it to unflinching rationalists, however, to draw explanation and system from under the wreckage of the reasoning intellect. It might seem futile today, but not too long ago a learned physician, Doctor Dumas, diligently toiled to set the record straight in matters of saintly smells.[6] For instance, he showed by rigorous historical research that the miraculous effluvia that rose from the body of Saint Catherine of Ricci were due to an overdose of medication. Terbentine, an aromatic compound extracted from oil of turpentine, was for a long time a popular medicament; until recently it was widely prescribed as an expectorant. Dumas reconciled the terminal symptoms of Saint Catherine (she lost the ability to form urine), the witnesses' descriptions of the odor she emitted, and the evidence of the saint's meek submission to her physician's prescriptions, and concluded that she must have succumbed to terbentine intoxication.

It must not be supposed that odor as an aid to diagnosis is a thing of the past. As recently as 1983, a physician admonished professionals to regard their olfactory sense as an instrument for diagnosis, and listed in the prestigious *New England Journal of Medicine* some of the diseases that historically have been associated with specific odorous qualities. These include phenylketonuria, in which the urine has a musty, barny, wolflike scent, "like stale, sweaty locker-room towels"; maple syrup disease, a condition in which the odor is that of dried malts or hops; hypermethioninemia, wherein the odor detected is sweet, fruity, like rancid butter or boiled cabbage; diphtheria emanates a sweetish smell; yellow fever's scent is reminiscent of a butcher shop; scurvy is putrid; scrofula has the aroma of stale beer; typhoid fever smells like "fresh-baked brown bread"; and diabetic coma is acid-fruity.[7]

Dumas's conclusion that Saint Teresa of Avila was summoned to join her beloved spouse, our Maker, by diabetes mellitus requires a preliminary explanation of pathophysiology. It is well known that in diabetes mellitus the metabolism of sugars is disturbed. In the normal state, sugars are the main fuel that the body uses for energy, and insulin is the hormone that promotes this utilization. Insulin is deficient in the diabetic patient, and this causes fat to be used for energy, as occurs in starvation. Among the products of degradation of fat are volatile compounds called "ketone bodies," which may rise tenfold or more in the blood and body fluids during severe, uncontrolled diabetes. The elimination of ketone bodies accounts for a certain odor of acetone in the patient's breath. The specific qualities of the odor are difficult to describe (of "sour apples," it has been said, or *pommes aigrelettes* if the diagnostician is also a gourmet); all agree, however, that it is not an unpleasant smell.

Dumas analyzes the detailed records of the last days of Teresa's life and concludes in favor of diabetes as the cause of her demise. Quoting the trustworthy records of Sepúlveda, he reconstructs the events preceding her death: her busy, tiresome occupations after the founding of the convent at Burgos; her mortifications and fasts, followed by progressive tiredness; and the exhausting trip from Medina del Campo to the village of

Penaranda, where coma and death supervened. The "sweet
odor" that the saint had exhaled became so prominent in the
room where her body was kept that the windows had to be
opened. Days after her remains had been buried, a habit that
she had worn, the bed on which she had rested, and even a
basin in which she had washed retained the "sweet odor of
Teresa." Although the characteristics of the scent were not
described, and the exaggerations of religious fervor had to be
discounted, the details of the narrative accorded well with the
hypothesis that decompensated diabetes had been the postern
through which the saint had proceeded to her deserved
recompense.

Oh, the arrogant materialism of "clinical noses"! Not content
with trying to diagnose sundry ailments through acrid, pungent,
sweetish, or fetid odors, they must still destroy the idea that
holiness supersedes natural law, and that a suave, persistent
aroma issuing from a human body is a miraculous occurrence.
As the caterpillar quits its chrysalis transformed into a brilliantly
colored butterfly, so, too, when the soul extends its wings and
flies heavenward an astonishing transmutation was believed to
have been wrought in the whole bodily economy. The body
was thought to become fresher, stronger, more supple as virtue
reconcentrated; and when saintliness was reached, modesty and
virtue oozed as vapor, imparting to perspiration the qualities of
perfume.

To this poetical interpretation the good doctor opposes the
idea that the odor of sanctity was due to ketone bodies, chiefly
aceto-acetic acid and β-hydroxybutyric acid. To state it briefly,
the odor of sanctity has the formula $CH_3 COCH_2 COOH$. Is
there nothing sacred anymore?

On Bad Odors

Of the malignancy of some odors little needs to be said. You know the stubborn quality of a disagreeable smell. It assails you when you least expect it. One day, you stroll casually outdoors, and there it is: the repugnant companion of a revolting object. It hovers invisible over a dead and decomposed animal, a piece of carrion, or a heap of excrement. You turn away from the repelling sight, but it is no use: the smell has taken hold of you and does not leave. Or else it diffuses relentlessly, from unseen origins. For it is not necessary to associate visual image and olfaction; the latter has a presence of its own, and such power as can persecute you, and harass you, like a maddening obsession.

Perhaps you encounter it first upon turning a corner: a whiff that lashes you in the face and grabs you by the throat. You turn around and retrace your steps, but it is still with you. You quicken your pace, but its presence seems to have smeared the inside of your nasal cavity. You run, and run, and sharply wend your way over walls, around corners, across doors. There. It seems that you have left it behind you. But then, once more, the emanation suffuses the air: it is with you.

It may happen that you change clothes, and still perceive it; that you immerse yourself in the bathtub, and still detect it; or that you douse yourself under a shower—without ridding yourself of its presence. It may be that you spray the air with the contents of a pressurized can of disinfectant, or uncover a solid bar of deodorant, or even sprinkle cologne, or perfume, over your own skin. And then, underneath the disinfectant, across the deodorant, and through the perfume, the repugnant odor again makes its presence felt. Is there anything more terrifying than this malignant, obsessive immanence?

It stays with you, it possesses you, like an incubus. And mark that its presence not merely incommodes you, but brands you, stigmatizes you. You become an outcast: like too visible a scarlet letter sewn on your clothes, or a number tattooed on your skin, the stamp of a repulsive odor proclaims your undesirability, identifies you as a misfit of the social order. Professor Nencki, at the time when he was immersed in his studies of the chemical compound skatole, a prototype of substances with a putrid odor, was asked to leave the reading room of the Museum Society of Bern. Likewise, Peter Griess, going home from his laboratory after a day of arduous scientific toil and experimentation with the chemical compounds of putrefaction, was unkindly received by fellow passengers in an omnibus in Burton. We can imagine the composed, generally phlegmatic bus riders, nervously directing sidelong glances at the organic chemist; then, removing themselves gradually from the offensive passenger; until this one, surrounded by an empty space as wide as the conditions of the crowded bus permitted, and irked by the hostile whispering, exclaimed, "Ladies, it is not what you think!"[8]

Just as a good odor seems to affirm life and to hearten its perceivers, so a bad odor discourages, and detracts from life's enjoyment. Its harm is proportionate to its intensity. Indeed, an ancient belief held that a bad odor, if strong and offensive, could kill us in a short time. An engaging author of centuries past, Doña Oliva Sabuco, gave it as proven that sudden death was an occupational hazard of latrine cleaners, and that "many horses have been found dead by the stink of dung moved about in the stables, to clean them."[9] Naïve, at best, were the examples with which she buttressed her argument: that those who are given smoke during interrogation, "to make them yield," may die from "nefarious odors," or that bees are prompt to abandon their hidden treasure when smoked out by honey-seekers. But well into the Age of Reason and throughout last century's scientific revolution, the belief in the lethal power of unclean, foul air went unchallenged.

Nor was there a dearth of confirmatory occurrences. "Mephitic gas," or pestilential, noxious emanations, lurked all around and could strike at any moment. An example was the sudden death of a gardener at the hospital in the French town of Béziers, struck dead while sprinkling the garden with water contaminated by the sewers. Or the death of the owner of a Parisian cellar that became filled with the fetid stench of decomposing corpses, when the crypt of an adjoining cemetery crumbled under the weight of too many burials.[10] Death haunts the infected sites, which number myriads in the cities. The refuse of markets; the dejecta of animals and human beings; the pestiferous effluvia from hospitals and slaughterhouses; a thousand sources of foul and putrid odors diffuse their threatening, invisible poisons as villages grow into huge metropolises. Scientific experiments contemporaneous with early urban growth, showing that small animals invariably die when enclosed in hermetically sealed glass containers, did more than underscore dramatically the vital nature of gas components. To a public unaccustomed to think in terms of analytical chemistry, such experiments meant that deadly miasmas constantly arose from living bodies, just as they did from dead and decomposing bodies. Hence the perilous quality of stagnant air. Hence the salutary effects of open spaces and ventilation. The first attempts at

sensible city planning were not inspired by aesthetic considerations but by public health concerns; and foremost among these
was fear of the malignant effluvia sent forth by crowded human
beings, their dejecta, their helter-skelter markets with decomposing hoarded produce, and their chaotically arrayed habita-
tions. Parisian planners with originality and foresight envisioned
(but never actually built) huge fans, like windmills, actuated by
the flowing waters of the river Seine, and placed at street corners.
Their sempiternally rotating blades were to send off beneficent
air currents that would scatter away all the overhanging sickly
and fetid vapors.

Organic decomposition elicited the greatest apprehension.
The rotting of dead animals, the putrefaction of human corpses,
and the gangrene of human parts were feared as great dangers.
Above all, stagnant air was to be avoided. Architectural styles
of hospitals, markets, and slaughterhouses were influenced by
these fears. Provisions were made for corridors in hospitals, or
adequate exits in buildings where it was urgent to facilitate the
disposal of decaying matter. The dead, however, constantly
threatened the living from unplanned, dangerously crowded
cemeteries. At length, these had to be refashioned: the dead
had to be "evicted." And this had to be done without disturbing
their peace, or offending the religious sentiments of the living.

In Paris, the "movers" set to work at night, on April 7, 1786.
Their picks and shovels poked the earth until they hit the feared
remains. Out came earth-covered skulls, mandibles, and fragments of thoracic walls with their evenly spaced ribs, now
balustrades for maggots. Huge carts were loaded with the mass
of half-decomposed parts, and went rumbling through the streets
toward the new cemetery, remote from the densely inhabited

city. As they wheeled the gruesome cargo over hilly cobblestoned streets, the trepidation sometimes caused an ill-preserved anatomical part to fall to the ground. A large retinue of cowled monks and their assistants followed, picking up the debris, intoning prayers, singing hymns, and uttering reiterative litanies. The whole operation was done by the light of torches held by the pious processionists. A solemn, fearful spectacle they offered, as their shadows projected on the walls, their monotonous prayers resounded along the way, and the heavy air, trapped in the canyons of the narrow streets, became filled with an unbearable stench. Nevertheless, this operation had to be repeated several times, as it was impossible to mobilize the entire army of the deceased in a single night.

Mephitic gases still surround and envelop mankind. True, we have today advanced sewage systems, processing plants, water-cleansing technology, and recycling stations that transform refuse into useful and tidy objects. But the balance is precarious: underneath the polished surface, filth accrues; and our enhanced powers of production only multiply the generation of unclean and deadly litter. Cervantes created the mad Licenciado Vidriera, a lunatic who fancied himself made of glass and lived in mortal fear of hard, moving objects and loud noises that might, he thought, crack him. A writer of our day could well imagine a man developing an olfaction-centered psychosis, becoming uniquely sensitive to gaseous stimuli and mortally scared of the effects of bad smells. It would be easy to depict this personage as growing ever more alienated in our technological midst; ever more pained by conscious awareness of the massive filth that accumulates in modern cities. The exhaust fumes of motorized vehicles and the motley emanations of crowds would set him in agony. To tread on beautiful lawns, to saunter in the fields, or in the gardens, would afford him no solace. For he would sense that the fresh greensward is but a thin film, under which exists an immense netherworld of slime, injurious gases, worm-ridden dead animals, man-made pipes that conduct waste, and the decomposing cadavers of the generations that preceded us on the crust of this deceptively bucolic earth.

Odors Evocative and Erotic

An anecdote told by chroniclers, over whose veracity I would not wager, has it that the French king Henry III, during certain festivities that celebrated the betrothal of Henry of Navarre and Margaret of Valois, dried his face with a garment of Marie of Cleves that was moist with her perspiration. If the event really took place, charity would compel us to hope that the lady exuded a sweet fragrance and the aroma of flowers, as did the saints; or at least that she conformed to that wholesome disposition that the good ancient poets attributed to desirable women—namely, that of having almost no scent at all. As Plautus put it, "A woman smells good who smells not at all" (*Mulier tum bene olet, ubi nihil olet*. Mostellaria, Act I, sc. iii, 117); and Montaigne, with his usual zesty insight, added that good scents ought to be like good actions, the best of which always course unannounced and unperceived.

Imagine the circumstances. Having conceived a juvenile passion for Marie of Cleves (despite indications of his aberrant sexuality), he comes upon a sweaty shirt, or a jerkin, of his beloved. He presses his face against the garment, and aspirates deeply. Let cynics smile, and the squeamish step back, cringing, at the grossness of this act. Those in love will readily perceive the symbolism: an object is greatly valued because it has existed in propinquity with the beloved. To hold it out for contemplation would not be enough; to touch it, though pleasing, would be less than satisfying. The object must be palpated, held out to view, and then, if its physical characteristics allow it, the lover's face must be buried in it, while voraciously aspirating through the nose the invisible, cherished reality of which it is imbued. Through the nose, precisely: such is the absorptive route that our elemental nature decrees. The Trobriand Islanders, like other preliteral peoples, were convinced that magic, to be maximally effective, must gain entrance through the nose.[11] This is why their love potions were made over mint and aromatic herbs, and carried about in odoriferous containers.

A profound cause underlies this behavior. Olfaction is a most intimate manner of knowing the external world. Vision and hearing are indirect ways of perceiving things. It is not the objects themselves that we see and hear: it is vibrations, waves, electromagnetic cyclic disturbances impressing our sensorium. It is otherwise with olfaction, during which the very substance of the perceived object must come in contact with our receptive organ. An infinitesimally small alluvion constantly occurs: molecules break off the surface of odorous materials—all early scientists marveled at the capacity of scented bodies to send off detectable particles without an apparent decrease in weight— and these staggeringly minute portions of the object become perceptible as they accumulate on the surface of our nasal tissue.

Here, close contact is indispensable for olfaction to occur. The odoriferous molecules are carried in eddies of inspired air to the roof of the nasal cavity, where an area no greater than

200–400 mm² is covered by olfactory receptor cells (the olfactory surface is increased, however, by hairlike prolongations, or cilia, of these cells); the slightest barrier interposed between odorant and perceiver would suppress the odorous reaction. The physiology of olfaction is incompletely understood, but the interaction is known to require very close contact between odorant molecules and the membrane of receptor cells. The "stereochemical" theory, still current today, proposes that the odors of substances are due to the size and shape of molecules: olfactory cells presumably contain receptor sites of definite shapes and dimensions, into which substances of appropriate molecular configuration may "fit," like the pieces of a puzzle.[12] Molecules able to secure a good "fit" would have one of the primary odors. It has also been proposed that the membranes of receptor cells are actually "punctured" and penetrated by the odorant molecules, thereby initiating the nervous impulse that is carried as an odoriferous message to the brain.[13] Whatever its exact mechanism, olfaction seems to express a relation of extraordinarily close proximity between perceiving self and odorant nonself. It is as if objective reality not merely abutted our sensitive faculty but actually merged with it.

Perhaps this is why olfaction has so powerful an evocative force. Pleasant odors almost always evoke a certain desire, or a yearning, which is rarely fulfilled. Leopardi remarked that often we are driven to inhale with great strength, as if to assuage the unsatisfaction, or to complete the pleasure, without ever quite succeeding. In fragrant foods, and in foods that are good to eat, odor often overcomes flavor; and the latter rarely measures up to the expectation that odor had made us conceive. "For if you carefully observe," wrote Leopardi, "you will agree that upon smelling such things we are overtaken by the desire, which comes to us sometimes in life, of plunging into, of becoming one with that source of pleasure; this compels us to place the food in our mouth, and having done so we are disappointed."[14] We are similarly excited when we smell a fragrant liquid: upon inhaling, the desire to drink it is aroused, but no amount of swills will quench the yearning. More than an ordinary strength of character is requisite to appease olfaction-kindled desire. Hence, the showy, baroque feats of renunciation of Saint Romualdo. This valorous "soldier of Christ" engaged the enemy, temptation, with temerity, not just with courage. When in the midst of his fasts the pleasures of the palate distressed him, he ordered the savory delicacy he had imagined immediately prepared and brought to him. He then held the dainty preparation close to his mouth and his nose, but "took only the odor [*solum captans odorem*], saying: 'O throat, throat, how sweet and soft and delectable this food would taste to you; but, woe to you! you shall never taste it.' And saying this, he sent the dish back to the kitchen."[15]

On purely theoretical grounds, a sound reasoner might have deduced a prominent role in sexuality for olfaction, a sense so evocative, so intimate and suggestive. This, indeed, is borne out by experience. In the breeding season, the air is heavy with scents that quicken the mating instinct of countless species. Theophrastus believed that even the rugs or mats made of goatskins emanated an odor in this season.[16] Modern science has known, since 1950, that chemically defined substances, known as pheromones, influence the mating behavior of insects. Since the initial investigations, it has become clear that male insects are lured to the female, sometimes for distances in excess of two miles, via perception of scents owed to pheromones. That the action of these substances is olfactory was inferred from the extremely small concentration sufficient to produce an observable response in the male. A few picograms (one picogram is a millionth of a millionth of a gram, or 10^{-12} gram), or a few molecules of the compound, are enough to set the male "excited and wildly flapping its wings," as stated in a journalist's colorful account of the typical reaction of wing-raising and rapid motions considered an indication of some insects' mating behavior, and thus a sensitive method of bioassay. A millionth of a picogram (10^{-18} gram!) of "Bombycol," a pheromone of the silkworm moth *Bombyx mori*, in one cubic centimeter of solvent was enough to instantaneously transform unconcerned, indifferent silkworm moths into solicitous males, eager for breeding.

For female insects, individual success in amorous emprise is often linked to the ability to secrete pheromones through the lower abdominal parts. The queen bee, armed with a formidable set of powerful mandibles, presents sex attractants through her mouth, an arrangement that perhaps offers a horrid fascination to the drone, lover and victim at the same time. During experiments at the University of Wisconsin using female pine sawflies (*Dipiron similis*) as baits, individual disparities in sex appeal were strikingly revealed. In some traps no males were caught, but female-baited traps on the average caught about one thousand males apiece. One extraordinary female—may her name endure in whatever annals may record the prowesses of six-legged seductresses—attracted eleven thousand males in eight days, and this in spite of the trivial fact that for the last three days she had been quite dead![17]

No such strength may be expected of human pheromones, assuming these were identified, synthesized, and marketed. The $3.5 billion U.S. industry of perfumery dreams of the day when volatile substances of comparable impact will be bottled for human consumption; a smell of these odorants presumably would lay low most men and women's principled circumspection, and topple the social order—all in one whiff. The reader would do well to note that there are some grounds for this disquieting forecast. Recently, the popular press gave prominent coverage to the work of Philadelphia researchers whose findings at the Monell Chemical Senses Center and the University of Pennsylvania further affirmed the importance of pheromones in human sexual life.[18] A "male essence" (exquisite designation of noble philosophical lineage) was collected from sweaty pads that men had worn under the armpits. Extracts prepared from the underarm secretion were swabbed three times a week on the upper lips of seven women whose menstrual cycles were abnormal, being at least three days longer or shorter than the normal 29.5 days. Control subjects received an alcoholic solution minus the "essence," and the studies were performed with neither researchers nor subjects knowing whether alcohol or male preparation was being applied. By the end of the study period the women who received "male essence" had altered their menstrual cycles, which now approached the normal rhythm, optimal for fertilization to occur. A unique hormone, produced by one individual and exerting its effects upon another subject, i.e., a pheromone, was thought responsible for the observed effect.

As to the advertising claims of perfumery ("enriched with pheromones, scientifically proven to drive men wild!"), a modicum of skepticism seems warranted. Nor is a breakthrough needed to ensure the future of this formidable industry. Nose and sex are indissolubly joined by that primeval link that imparts to all our fundamental experience a kind of nasal repercussion, much like the oscillation of an untouched string that vibrates in synchrony, if not "in sympathy," with the one stroked. Nasal tissues seem immoderately sensitive to sexual hormones. Ancient and modern clinical observations document the existence of women in whom periodic nosebleeds are a form of vicarious menstruation. The connective tissue of the nasal mucosa, rich in vascular lakes, is prompt to react with engorgement (tumescence) and is highly sensitive to the action of sex hormones. It is strikingly similar, as histologists know, to erectile penile tissue. And if it is true that much incredible lore and fantastic speculation have arisen from purported sexual-nasal homologies and associations, it is also true that clinicians continue to encounter such pathological fare as "honeymoon rhinitis," in which the shock occasioned by a sudden surge of sex hormones becomes too much for a nasal mucosa formerly inured to more subdued stimulation.

Beyond what is purely physiological, sex and olfaction thrive in the deepest strata of the mind. Both lie at the core of the psychic persona. Long before we attempted to recognize articulated sounds, or complex visual patterns, smell and sex were preeminent in relational life. Olfaction and sexuality became engraved in the oldest part of the brain (in evolutionary terms), the archipallium, whereas the intellect, on which the pride of our species is made to rest, appeared much later. Long, long ago, when our remote ancestors partly supported their unseemly gait with their hands; when they migrated in great nomadic

herds enveloped in clouds of dust, pressed on by dwindling food
and the fear of menacing beasts; when grunts and snarls formed
all human discourse: that was the time when olfaction and sex
were cast as sustaining pillars of all future human cerebration.
It was then that a whiff of air would tell fellow herd member
from alien and potential foe. And it was then that the sniff of
hirsute females in heat, whom our remote forebears held in
common, excited the males of the herd to that congress that
is now deemed an act of love, but which was then not much
different from the rabid encounters of predators that daily
bloodied the hostile plains.

These remote beginnings do not escape the notice of the
modern perfume industry. Commercial appeals are made ad-
visedly, in full cognizance of the fact that to address our nose
is to address our deepest self. It is not surprising that a high
executive of Flavors and Fragrances Company of New York,
interviewed on television, described the unflagging toils by which
researchers at his firm endeavor to recreate an odor of "new
car"; a more exotic one of "eighteenth-century London" (although, if those perfumers and advertisers cared to read the
writings of Londoners of that era, I am afraid the effort to
reproduce this scent would seem ill-advised); and still another
one, on which vast sums of money were being spent, the odor
of "sun-dried clothes."[19]

As odorant molecules touch, and perhaps wound, our nasal
mucosa, messages are conveyed to the phylogenetically most
ancient region of the brain. Little wonder that memories are
stirred and yearnings are awakened in a way that no other sense
can duplicate. A familiar landscape; the long-forgotten flavor of
a spicy dish; the very experience of childhood: all may be

summoned into conscious awareness at the promptings of smell. May the chemist succeed in trapping the elusive scents in a flask, as Aladdin trapped the genie in a bottle. For if all must be forgotten—and it is appointed that *all* must be forgotten—scents are the only scraps of reality that I should care to retain. Sounds and sights, for all their splendor, lack the elementary immediacy, the molecular contact that lends odors their unexampled evocative force. When the features of a loved face will have blurred; when pitch and inflection of a cherished voice will no longer beckon distinctly; what vivid pleasure, then, to open a flask and inhale the fundamental, irreducible reality of an odor. Oh, for the odor of the absent one!

SIGHT

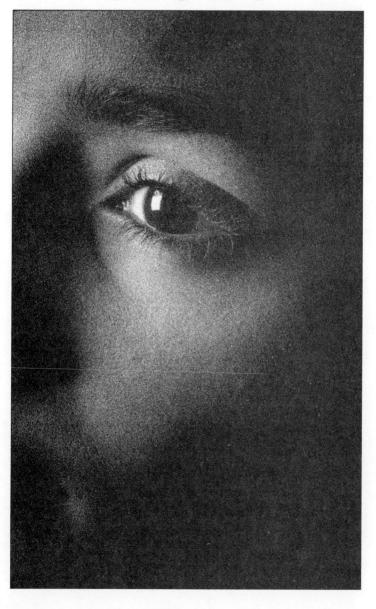

Ocular Surroundings

THAT THE EYES are "windows of the soul" is a poetical allusion often credited to Leonardo da Vinci. Yet, even assuming the truth of that illustrious parentage, the metaphor seems now trite and ineffective. Poll, if you would, the well-informed: their vote is likely to go for the idea that emotion has better indicators elsewhere. Where? Sophistication in physiology, be it ever so modest, suggests a wide range of choices: the adrenal glands, whose brisk output signals fight or flight; the nasal mucosa, whose swift engorgement with blood the observer may rightly consider a sensitive gauge of emotional tension; or perhaps the stomach, whose proximity to the heart betokens, in Van Helmont's old view, the ability to receive the full impact of the heart-generated "passions"—and whose acid secretion and spasmodic reactions remind us, at every jostle and trample of contemporary life, that emotion may be denoted most keenly at sites far removed from the organs of visual perception.

Still, one may argue for the expressive supremacy of the eye, be it ever so timorously. One could say that ocular expressiveness is acknowledged by all to be strictly a matter of appearances; that if we confine our canvassing to the face, it becomes evident that the eye is, of all facial features, inherently the most expressive. For even animals, according to popular belief, look man "in the eye" when desirous of guessing his intentions. Yet this very assertion would not pass uncontested. Its detractors would point out that the concerned quarry searches not for the pupils of the hunter. For it is not the eye globe, itself relatively

set and inexpressive, that translates our inner agitations; it is
the eye's complex surroundings—eyebrows, eyelids, skin
creases, and frontal and periocular muscles—that compose facial
expression. And we would be hard put to deny the strong
evocative power and subtle magic of periocular structure.

Consider the eyebrow. In man, this coppice of hair is expressive to a degree unmatched in the animal kingdom. Raised
in surprise, converging in concentration, and slanting or spreading out in bewilderment, the eyebrow signals with its motions
assent, dissent, sternness, and shock. Four emotions the ancients
linked with the brow: sorrow, mirth, pity, and severity (*tristitiae,
hilaritatis, clementiae, severitatis index*). One passion, however, was
said by Pliny (*Nat. Hist.*, Book 11, Ch. 50) to make its permanent
abode in the eyebrow. This is pride, whose nature is by definition
"supercilious." And to explain the curious phenomenon the
ancient naturalist tells us that pride, though born in the heart,
at once rises and hangs tenaciously from the brow: *in corde
nascitur, huc subit, hic pendet.* Does it not seem an eminently
reasonable account? Pride is the one passion that cannot be
made to suffer a relatively lowly or inferior birthplace. It must
climb at once, and finding no loftier position in the expressive
face than the brow, it settles there, for only there its vainglorious
nature may be contented with being the sole occupant.

It is also true that the countenance is modified by the eyelid,
this movable, skin-covered curtain that rises or falls between
the external world and the perceiving consciousness. Pliny could
not have failed to remark on the outstanding examples. Thus,
he tells us that the emperor Gaius had staring eyes; that Claudius
Caesar's were frequently bloodshot and had a fleshy gleam at
the corners; and that Augustus had gray eyes like those of horses,

the whites larger than normal for human beings, owing to his often being angered by curious onlookers who stared at him too long. In our day, panegyrists of the Ayatollah Khomeini's hawklike mien are not above basing his regal and imposing appearance wholly upon his eyes: dark and fiery, deep set, and framed by hirsute black eyebrows and "hoodlike" eyelids.

There is, however, a curious point offered to the analyst of eye structure: the arrangement and disposition of the eyelid is not the same in every race. The prototypical Asiatic upper eyelid extends down smoothly to its termination at the eyelash-rimmed border. The Westerner's, in contrast, is interrupted by a transverse fold that creates upper and lower regions, above and below this fold. The Asiatic upper eyelid, having a greater amount of fatty tissue compared to Caucasians, is displayed like a slightly puffy, unbroken, full drape. Leaner of preorbital tissues, its Western counterpart evinces the effect of muscle fibers that attach to the underside of the palpebral skin. It is the retraction of these muscle fibers that creates the transverse fold.

These anatomical peculiarities may seem trivial. But no detail of our bodily structure is without effect upon our ideas, and hence without impress upon our lives. Roland Barthes[1] realized this when he attributed the origin of two different popular mythologies to the shape of the eyes in the East and the West. The thinner (and folded) upper eyelid of Westerners outlines the spheroidal ocular globe which it covers. Accordingly, the effect produced is a "sculptoric" one, of mass and volume. And this is why "the Western eye is subject to a whole mythology of the soul, central and secret, whose fire, sheltered in the orbital cavity, radiates towards a fleshy, sensuous, passional exterior. . . ." In the West, indeed, folklore, tradition, and literature invite us to look "deep into the eyes" of others, to gaze through the "windows" of the soul we wish to understand. It is otherwise in the East, for the Asiatic eye, lacking a fold in the structures that drape it, appears smooth and level with the rest of the face. And thus the Oriental eye, by virtue of its morphology, "cannot be read 'in depth,' i.e., according to its axis of inwardness; its model is not sculptural but scriptural: it is a flexible, fragile, close-woven stuff (silk, or course), simply and as though immediately calligraphed in two lines."

Two lines: a curved upper one for the eyebrow, and a slanting, single inferior line for the palpebral fissure. Roland Barthes, for whom life was identical to a grandiose writing process (or, to phrase it differently, life was reducible to the fundamental mechanisms that control writing), could not have ignored this metaphor: the Oriental face was not "made," but was "written." It was written as Oriental script, with Oriental writing tools. The slit of the eye is traced by a single rapid stroke of the brush, starting at the inner corner, the medial canthus, and swiftly extending outward. The pressure of the tracing is gradually diminished, so that the line becomes progressively thinner, until it ends up in a pointed outer tail, a nimbly traced, evanescent, gradually disappearing outer tip. The upper curved line is the brow, and between the two lines the calligrapher leaves an unwritten blank space.

Opposed to this metaphoric conception of the fashioning of the Oriental eye, human folly devised the concrete means for its defacement. The process is based on the perverted aesthetics of "Westernization." It is accomplished by a combination of neurotic dissatisfaction in the patient and a suspect officiousness in the surgeon. The operation, known as blepharoplasty, creates a fold in the unfolded upper eyelid. It is by no means rare: a Singapore surgeon reported more than five thousand cases from his individual experience.[2] The procedure aims to achieve the "sculptoric" effect of which Barthes spoke, but is itself unmistakably scriptural: the writing brush is a scalpel, and the strokes are as difficult and exacting as those of calligraphy, an art that demands the utmost concentration from its practitioners. At exact distance, measured with calipers from anatomical landmarks, the calligrapher-surgeon traces his flourishes: it is not possible to erase. The written character is read in the cutaneous scar that the scalpel/brush leaves in the wake of its motions. The intent is to write the character that stands for "Western eye," but imperfections in the execution may render unwanted pictographs, such as those that stand for "eyes asymmetrical," "bizarre gaze," or, in the worst possible outcome, the character that stands for "blindness."

Fascination

If truth be told, periocular structures are merely externals. They are but the foil against which the eye shines brighter. For it is still the eye, at the center of these wrappings, underneath mantles and protective awnings, that "makes silence eloquent," as Addison wrote, and is capable of bestowing life to every part of us. Nor is this just poetical metaphor. Using videotapes, researchers have shown that the attention of infants, as early as a few weeks after birth, is fixed upon the eyes of the mother.[3] Among the mother's facial features are some that vie for the attention of her nursing infant: the lips are mobile and may be painted red; the nose juts out; and the teeth are flittingly exposed. Nevertheless the attention of the infant is preferentially riveted upon the mother's eyes. It is thus not entirely inaccurate to say that the "power of the gaze" is objectively documented. Something in the eye is tended across space and bathes us, envelops us, and exerts its sway upon us.

Until the nineteenth century, vision was explained by the "emanation" theory. Light was thought to consist of a kind of stream of particles emitted by the object seen. But the eye itself was long thought to be the source of another emanation ("visual spirit" was its appealing name during the Middle Ages), and vision was understood to result from the collision of particles from these two sources.[4] Today's interpretation of vision speaks of a unidirectional flow. Whether made of electromagnetic waves or other forms of energy, a million images filter across the pupil. The universe made light flows through this tiny aperture before striking the retina, which is but filmy brain substance turned inside out and molded into a cuplike receptacle. From here, on both sides, the current of energy travels inwardly to some central brain station wherein the flow of energy is at last transformed into perceived image. Nowhere in the modern theory of vision do we find support for the deep and abiding belief, ever thriving in the popular mind, that energy sparked in the brain's recondite recesses travels contrary to the visual impulses and emerges through the pupils.

Yet, the popular fantasy almost never arises out of wanton disregard for objectivity. The foundation of magic and superstition is not strictly fanciful: the observations are "correct," but the deductions are false. Thus, to explain the power of the gaze as a function of forces emerging through the pupil, much is made of narratives that attest to the might of the eyes: a resolute glance from a hero suffices to stir a whole army into action; and the look from a mother's eyes stops cold the ferocious beast about to devour her young. Ancient chroniclers profusely added to such documentation. Of twenty thousand gladiators in the training school of the emperor Gaius, only two had eyes that did not blink when faced by some threat, and were, therefore, invincible. During the principate of Claudius, a Gaetulian shepherd decountenanced a lion that charged at him by flinging his cloak over its eyes, and thus performed the incredible feat of nullifying its awful rage. Lysimachus, shut up in a cage with a lion by order of Alexander, resorted to the same trick and succeeded in strangling it. The unanimous conclusion of early observers is that leonine rage, like human passion, is at least partly channeled through the eyes, and thus may be opposed effectively by counteracting vision.

It seemed immediately obvious that the power of the eye may be of a wholly negative kind. Such is *oculus fascinus*, the "evil eye." Nicolas Oresme, bishop of Lisieux in the fourteenth century, defined fascination using the comprehensive language of science: "It is the impression of suffering or infection, made on a human being or another animal by the glance of another man or animal." Note that the evil eye is not exclusively human: a wolf, if it sees a man first, renders him speechless. A rational soul is not indispensable to the exercise of the malignant visual impression; however, plants or inanimate objects cannot exert it. Medieval philosophy offers a solution to these riddles. The soul is divided into compartments of different hierarchical status. Although the evil eye must always work through the instrumentality of a soul, it is the sensitive, not the rational or vegetative soul that must be operative. Medieval scholars may disagree on the details of such theorizing, but are in perfect agreement as to the inherent malignancy of human eyes kindled by passion. When lust seethes in the eye; when envy festers behind the gaze, or hatred in the heart of the gazer; then it is that the fiery rays that shoot through the pupil are at their most dangerous. Envy, especially, is to be feared. Francis Bacon echoed the universal distrust of envious glances, which persists among many people in our enlightened age: "There seemeth to be acknowledged in the act of Envy an ejaculation or irradiation of the eye. Nay, some have been so curious as to note that the times when the stroke or percussion of an envious eye doth most hurt are when the party envied is beheld in glory or triumph, for that sets an edge upon envy; and besides, at such times the spirits of the person envied do come forth most into the outward parts, and so meet the blow."[5] Of all superstitions, this is perhaps the longest lasting and most widespread. The nearly universal custom of veiling brides (or all women, as in Islam) apparently originated from the persuasion that ardent desire, lust, or envy can infuse the gaze with influences harmful to the person or object coveted.[6]

Théophile Gautier exploited the ancient superstition's rich lore in his masterful short story "Jettatura."[7] The protagonist, possessor of the deplorable gift of the evil eye, is a young French nobleman, Paul d'Aspremont. He is introduced in the story as an aristocrat of grand and distinguished bearing. This is a departure from folkloric tradition, in which the fascinator is, as a rule, ugly: not only capable of causing misfortune, but actually attempting to rid himself of illnesses and deformities that afflict him, and of which he often succeeds in freeing himself by a mysterious form of transference that passes these ills on to other people. Didymus warned against those who have hollow, pitlike, sunken eyes, and who emit a disagreeable odor; women were generally believed to possess more power of fascination than men, but the young and beautiful, according to various sources, were less apt to inflict serious illnesses than withered crones. In Gautier's short story, d'Aspremont is described as possessing noble features but nevertheless having a certain disharmony of expression. Individually considered, each of his facial features would seem comely and attractive. But somehow, in combination, they integrate a repelling whole. As it sometimes happens that an unskilled artist gives to a portrait the finest nose, the noblest brow, and the most perfect eyes he is capable of rendering, and yet the finished portrait is distinctly inferior to each of its component parts, so in the case of d'Aspremont the facial features seem not to go naturally together, and this disunity results in a facial appearance that strikes the observer as bizarre and unsettling.

D'Aspremont has come to Naples to visit his fiancée, who sojourns there upon medical advice. His arrival is remarked upon by the local people with a sense of apprehension and uneasiness. His reddish hair, steely gray eyes, and extremely pale complexion, joined to the ineffable disharmony of the face, mark him as the bearer of ill omens. Add to this several chance occurrences that take place in coincidence with the visitor's disembarkment—when the sea seems calm, a large wave capsizes the boat of porters who ferry the luggage to the harbor; the coachman who transports the travelers to the hotel falls from his seat while looking back to answer the foreigner—and you have all the necessary conditions to persuade the people of Naples that their visitor is no common tourist but a possessor of *il fascino*, the power to harm another person by a mere glance, without need to come in contact with his victim, or, indeed, of any other ministration.

Woe to those suspected to noxious visual power! They will become the outcasts of the community, blamed for misfortunes, dreaded by all, and rejected even by their friends and relatives. D'Aspremont is to find out that to be a *jettatore* is, in fact, a tragic destiny. It is an incurable malady. Not a state brought upon oneself through one's own actions, but purely the sad lot of fate, the mighty blow of a dark destiny that strikes at random. And just as bodily illness recognizes no rank, and spares not the rich and the socially exalted, so one is born a *jettatore* and remains one for life, regardless of one's desperate efforts to prevent it. D'Aspremont sees himself turning into such a victim. People flee from his proximity. His appearance at a social event is always received with fear, for the roof may collapse, or the food may become poisoned, or some other disaster may wreck the celebration and hurt the guests. Therefore, he must never figure in the list of guests; his presence must be avoided at all costs.

In Paris, in his familiar surroundings, D'Aspremont would have laughed at this situation. He would have shrugged off the suggestion of his ocular injuriousness as a coarse superstition, a sample of dismal ignorance incredibly persisting into the modern era. But the collective attitude that prevails in the Naples of the narrative tinctures his ideas with gloomier shades. Pedestrians step to the opposite sidewalk when they chance to encounter him on the street. Infants are shielded from his glances, for everyone knows that the child would catch the croup, a rheumy eye, smallpox, or worse if looked at by a

fascinator. Through the accomplished craft of Gautier the story-
teller, we hear the imprecations shouted behind d'Aspremont's
back; we see the fear on the face of credulous women as the
Frenchman approaches (pregnant women, above all, must be
careful to avoid him, for his piercing glances may provoke the
birth of infants weak, stillborn, or afflicted with monstrosities);
the bundles of garlic still hung behind doors, to protect the
household from his malignant gaze; and the hands with extended
index and little finger, all the other fingers flexed and enclosed
by the thumb, the gesture of horns, or *mano cornuta*, believed
to stave off the injurious emanation that flows from the eyes
of the fascinator.

In an enervating atmosphere of unwholesome heat, of shirts
that stick to the sweat-drenched torsos, of malaria (then prev-
alent in Naples), and of nearly universal adherence to irrational
belief, the mind of Paul d'Aspremont gradually assents to the
collective accusation. By dint of hearing protective invocations
in his presence, of seeing amulets hung round the neck of his
interlocutors, and sprigs of rue, vervain, or laurel displayed over
the doors that he is about to cross, he ends up believing in his
own power to injure with the eyes. He examines incidents of
his former life, that until then scarcely troubled him, and finds
them charged of a disturbing new significance. The death of his
mother shortly after he was born: was it not the consequence
of having brought him, a *jettatore*, into the world? In his childhood, d'Aspremont had been deeply troubled when he witnessed
the accidental fall of his best friend from a high tree branch,
during their games, causing his friend's permanent invalidism.
Now d'Aspremont wonders whether the fall had been an accident, or whether the tree branch had broken because he, a

fascinator, watched keenly the precarious evolutions of his friend. In vain does he pose such questions to himself. The answer, he believes, is in the *mano cornuta* that his interlocutors hide behind their backs, beneath their aprons, or inside their pockets, when they address him. And this grim answer, muttered, half-repressed, or brazenly shouted at him, is always the same: *"Jettatore! Jettatore!"*

Deluded into believing that he has the power to injure with his eyes, our man writhes in anguish as he sees the steady deterioration of his fiancée's health. He is convinced that his beloved is gradually consumed because his glances constantly sap her strength by what we might call "ocular vampirism." He confesses these fears to her, but she rebukes his arguments as the products of an overheated imagination stressed by hostile surroundings. What is more, with winsome, moving, virginal innocence, she owns that even if the awful suspicion were true, she would never leave him. She prefers to stay by his side, come what may.

In a collateral outgrowth of the main plot, d'Aspremont slays a rival who had publicly exposed him as a fascinator. The fatal contest is a duel with knives, during which both contenders band their eyes, as a concession to the code of honor that decrees that none should enjoy unfair advantage. Returned to the hotel still the prey of tempestuous emotions, excited by the recent bloody encounter, despondent over the imminent death of his beloved, overwhelmed by an irrational sense of guilt that finds reinforcement in the local prejudice against him, and deranged by alcoholic intake, the chief protagonist of the story, now on the verge of psychosis, blinds himself with hot irons abruptly thrust through his eyes. He recovers from the self-inflicted wounds in time to discover that his adored fiancée has just died. Although he is now completely blind, he finds his way to a high cliff by the sea, and ends his life by drowning in the Bay of Naples.

The modern reader is apt to react with impatience to this story, written very much in the spirit of the Romantic era that inspired it. The first half seems to announce the advent of comedy, but is followed by a very nineteenth-century melo-dramatic conclusion, with its inordinate love of the fantastic, and its depiction of exaggerated feelings, or of sentiment keyed several step-notes above today's acceptable harmony. But let us note that nothing in this fiction is "impossible," in the sense of being contrary to well-documented, reiterated observation. Belief in the evil eye is still widespread throughout the world. Physicians who practice in "ethnic" neighborhoods of large North American cities must reckon with it often; and affluence and education, as practitioners know well, do not always weaken its grasp. As to the episode of self-blinding, psychiatric experience attests to the terrible reality of such unspeakable assaults. The horror of it is almost too much to tell: a medical textbook devoted to eye-related psychic disturbances shows the close-up photo of a patient's eye from which only the eraser-tipped end of a wooden pencil emerges, while the entire shaft is buried in the eye globe; the text informs us that the victim was a deranged individual who appeared in the emergency room of a hospital, seized the pencil from the intern who was taking his clinical history, and plunged it straight into his eye. With clinical com-prehensiveness we are also told that the depicted attempt at self-blinding failed, as the pencil's tip reached deep into the orbit but narrowly missed the optic nerve, and function was eventually restored.[8]

Fascination as Clinical Syndrome

Upon such facts, the hideous together with the quaint, rests the concept of the centrality of eye and vision in the human personality. The "I," the self, is equated with the eye. And the expression of this fundamental conviction is ornate or simple in proportion as the personality is developed. At one extreme, a schizophrenic child, when asked to draw a human face, will sketch a large, fixed eye at the center of his inchoate, formless rendering. At the opposite extreme, pathology manifests itself in exotic turns of behavior. A Swiss patient described by Greenacre[9] appeared at the psychiatrist's office with his hat pulled down over his eyes and a handkerchief veiling his face to protect others from the look in his eyes, and himself from the harmful gaze of others. But these baroque clinical records are exceptional. Two forms of deviancy, exhibitionism and voy-eurism, are common enough to have become part of our regular, daily language. Both illustrate the medullary importance of vision in psychic life, and how, through the astonishing alchemy of disease, the individual consciousness is transmuted into an aggressive visual weapon, or into a passive seen object.

Exhibitionism was first described as a clinical entity by Lasègue, in 1877.[10] In the original communication, Professor Lasègue apologizes for introducing a neologism to designate this disease. He has no choice: heretofore the language of medicine has lacked words to name "the very numerous states intermediate between reason and madness," of which the described condition is most certainly an example. As for the standard, common language, ordinarily richer of denotative terms in this realm, its paucity in this case is just as apparent. Next, he embarks upon the phenomenological exposition of this deviancy, with case descriptions. A young man under thirty years of age, employed as the personal secretary of a prominent politician and belonging to a respected family, is arrested and charged with outrage to public morals. The authorities had received many complaints that an individual whose personal description closely coincided with that of the arrested suspect had provoked reiterated scandals inside churches, always at night. The young man appears suddenly in front of a woman absorbed in prayer in the semi-deserted sanctuary. Without pronouncing a word, he exposes his genitals, then quickly disappears into the shadows of the ambulatory. Great is the frustration of the law-enforcing agents: the large number of temples in the city rule out an effective surveillance. However, one evening, our man takes it into his head to strike inside the Church of St. Roch. He indulges his periodic fantasy in front of an old woman who is praying. The woman utters a scream. The watchman is alerted, and the offender is restrained in his flight with the help of irate parishioners.

Called to examine the accused, Lasègue must revise his own preconceptions. The suspect is not, as might be supposed, a moronic degenerate. Neither his position in the world nor his acquirements nor his personal gifts would have disbarred him from the assuagement of his sexual drive via legitimate, socially acceptable means. But interrogation sheds no light on the causes of his abnormal behavior. The detainee withdraws within himself, or explodes in tearful expressions of regret, or of remorse, never offering the slightest insight into his condition.

Additional cases come under Lasègue's scrutiny. However, new cases enlarge the phenomenological spectrum without clarifying the etiology. A sixty-five-year-old widower, the father of three who lives retired with his sister, is arrested by the police. He is in the habit of taking a daily morning stroll. Arriving at the iron gate of a girls' school at the time when the students are released for lunch break, he unbuttons his fly and exposes his genitals to the frightened schoolgirls who must parade in front of him while exiting through the gate. These embarrassing proceedings have acquired a ritualistic imprint. The old man follows the same route every morning, arrives at the site of his misdeed at a fixed time, deposits his ebony cane with silver handle always against the second iron bar to the left of the main door, and goes on to perform his indecent act. The bizarre scene has taken place at least ten times before the school authorities, apprised of the offense, forewarn the police and cause the apprehension of the wrongdoer.

Other examples are described, but the characteristics of individuals who manifest the disorder fall within no easily definable pattern. Some are intelligent, educated, and financially well-off; one of these, aware that a judicial inquest will bring dishonor to his family, emigrates to Belgium before his arraignment. Others are poor, infirm, or destitute; many among the latter are incarcerated and serve long prison terms. As to the general health of these patients, no common feature is evinced. They are either sound of body, or suffer various infirmities; either impotent, or capable of normal sexual activity; able to function in society, or hampered by obvious psychiatric dysfunction. Thus

Lasègue can only sketch the most general outline of the disorder. It is one marked by an episodic aberration of conduct whose distinguishing features are impulsiveness, periodicity, and instantaneousness. No organic lesion is discoverable. The patient is perfectly aware of the absurdity of his behavior and the dire consequences thereof, but is unable to restrain his impulse. The background upon which these striking episodes appear shares nothing in common with other forms of known mental illness. Rather, writes Lasègue, "as in the case of other intermittent maladies, such as malaria, gout, or hysteria, the fundamental derangement is subject to complete remissions" in the intervals between attacks.

More than a hundred years after this description, the amount of commentary and investigation is still disproportionate to the degree of basic understanding of the disorder. Lasègue's comparison strikes us as both quaint and outmoded, for we have learned much about diseases of intermittent clinical course. The patient with malaria continues to harbor the parasite between febrile episodes; the patient with gout is afflicted with a metabolic disturbance even when not in pain; and the patient with hysteria is not well between attacks, however difficult it may be to detect the disturbance. Our trust in biomedical science leads us to suppose that exhibitionism is one more instance of the "subtlety" of disease. The determinants of the affliction are too elusive for our present diagnostic means. The outrageous episodic conduct is the tip of the iceberg, we say to ourselves. There must be, underneath, a complex web of pathophysiology that awaits probing by keener and more penetrating diagnostic technologies than are now available. But together with these professions of confidence in the future of orthomolecular psy-

chiatry, a residue of skepticism tells us that eye-centered delusions will remain mysterious, that even the full inventory of
disturbed biochemistry will not wholly "explain" why vision
was made the central preoccupation.

The correlative malady is voyeurism: as the exhibitionist
wishes to be seen, the voyeur wishes to see. Only the urge to
see is, in the technical jargon of professionals, "overdetermined."
It is well known that the voyeur will go to extremes to satisfy
his craving. He will risk being arrested as a prowler, injured in
falling from trees, buildings, and other high observation posts,
afflicted with frostbite by remaining a long time in inclement
weather. Some have been shot at, even killed, when discovered
inside the house and confused with a burglar. What is it that
the voyeur wishes to see with this alarming unrestraint? Voyeurism, in a textbook definition, is the "exaggerated desire to
see, by stealth, a member of the opposite sex in some state of
undress, in the sexual act, or in the act of excretion," and this
desire is "so intense that it surpasses in importance the normal
sexual act." Ostensibly, the voyeur is the victim of an aberration
that confuses vision with genitalia. However, interrogation of
these patients makes it clear that the specific object of vision
that is sought may be unclear to the voyeur himself. Asked to
describe what the ideal voyeuristic scene would be that would
wholly satisfy him, a voyeur becomes puzzled, bewildered, and
cannot supply a concrete answer. One of them replied, "I don't
know . . . to see . . . to see more and more, I suppose . . .
more and more."

Mark the exotic trappings of this deviancy. The seeing must
be stealthy; the victim is to be caught unaware. A true voyeur
does not pay prostitutes to disrobe. Deliberate exposure of the

feminine body, as in a striptease, loses all its appeal. A patient confessed having attended stag shows and feeling indifferent to the spectacle; however, he was excited when he watched the show with half-closed eyelids: the glimpse taken through the inch-and-a-half space between blinds, stealthily, is infinitely more rewarding than unobstructed viewing, freely offered to the unhindered contemplation under a bright light.

It is thus easy to see that this deviancy is complex, far beyond the urge for simple visual perception. Clearly, at the bottom of the voyeuristic behavior there are elements of aggression, a need to seek out danger and to challenge the interdictions of society. In the common psychoanalytic interpretation, the voyeur uses the eye symbolically as an instrument of domination and punishment. A voyeur, describing his nightly sallies, said that he was usually deterred from carrying out his activities if he discovered a religious symbol, a cross or a star of David, displayed conspicuously on the window or in the bedroom he intended to watch. The spectacle of a family gathered in prayer would compel him to abandon his projects, and to look for another house, another target of his peeping. Only when he could imagine that the woman he peeped on was unchaste, brazen, or impious would he give himself freely to his bizarre and stealthy pleasure. Somehow, his visual organs were being used to punish the "shameless" woman who unwittingly exposed her nakedness.

When an exhibitionist provokes a visual experience, he does not intend to establish any form of personal relationship with the Other; his acts are never a pretext for closer contact. It is otherwise with the voyeur, who is impelled by aggressive or sadistic forces. A Peeping Tom may intentionally cough, or make a noise that will alert the person watched of his presence. For the realization that one is being exposed, unwillingly revealed, surprised in unwanted circumstances, is close to humiliation. In the often quoted article of Yalom,[11] voyeurs are described as potentially dangerous: in some cases, a Peeping Tom yielded to the unconscious urge to enter the house he prowled, not really knowing why he was doing it; in other cases, this act was followed by burglary; in still others, by sexual crime. Thus the voyeur, according to Yalom, is apt to "graduate" to more dangerous forms of behavior.

These clinical documents demonstrate, better than any amount of literary exegesis, the reality of the power of the gaze. The outreaching efficacy of vision is more than metaphoric: the gaze is sketched action. To look is to intend; in every glance there is the germ of an act. The eye *yearns* to grasp, to console, to imbibe, to eat, to petition, to warn, to undress, to caress, to fulminate, to confound, to kill. Valéry understood that visual perception resolves itself in pure intentionality: "How many babies if glances could impregnate! How many cadavers if glances could kill! The streets would be full of corpses and pregnant women."

So it is that deviancy teaches the reality of *oculus fascinus*. For if not fascination, what is it these patients look for? The voyeur hankers after the power to hurt through the gaze, the evil eye. Yet he is doomed to frustration; the natural limitations of sight sempiternally deny the satisfaction of desire. For this is the inherent irony of vision, that it reveals to us the enormity of the space beyond our bodies, and the shortness of our grasp. Visual perception makes it possible for us to yearn for what is beyond, and, *at the same time*, to realize that we cannot reach it. In vision, as in the other senses, lies an element of torture. Recall that the torture of Tantalus—condemned to suffer hunger and thirst while standing neck-deep in a pool of ever-receding water, and surrounded by delicious fruits just out of his reach—is as much an oral as it is a visual punishment. An appropriate punishment, considering that Tantalus had sinned doubly against the gods: by serving the flesh of his son at a banquet—an oral crime—and by divulging the secrets of the gods that he had learned illicitly—the crime of voyeurism, of which he stood indicted.

The exhibitionist's fantasy is anything but simple. On superficial examination it seems to be neither active nor aggressive. But upon slight reflection it becomes clear that his is a complex aggressiveness, a "passive aggression," which is a way of denoting a circular, coiled, or reflex passivity. His utmost pleasure consists not in seeing but in forcing others to see him. A profound though unconventional logic underlies his deviancy: by becoming pure passivity, he attains innocence. Moral codes are explicit in their prohibitions against evil acts. But the exhibitionist fancies that he "does nothing." He offers himself as an object of contemplation, as object-seen, as entity in total inactivity, and therefore free from blame. It is for others to worry about the consequences of their acts, or of the exercise of their visual function, the free play of the power of the gaze. So far as he is concerned, he is innocent. In the cross fire of glances that beam from every direction, he takes no part; he constitutes himself as a sacrificial victim, and his sense of culpability is accordingly expunged.

The exhibitionist's pleasure derives entirely from the sentiment that he attributes to others vis-à-vis himself. Is this not

an astonishing interaction? A pleasure that stems from the imaginary representation that one makes of the *fascination* that others
experience by being exposed to one's presence! Writers of fiction
could not have imagined a more curiously retroflexed inter-
dependence. It is for professionals to tell us what reaction the
exhibitionist imagines he produces in the Other—shock, horror,
desire?—or what sequels he anticipates—blows, appeals to the
police, seduction? What seems plain is that the exhibitionist
ultimately relates his desire to himself. His pleasure is thus
autoerotic, which is to say a regressive form of eroticism. Hence
its occurrence, albeit rarely, in women,[12] and the apparent
difficulty experienced by psychiatrists in distinguishing between
exhibitionism and narcissism.[13] At any rate, the exhibitionist is
also a being in quest of fascination. With unremitting drive he
searches for that mysterious "irradiation of the eye," that arcane
energy, not in his own but in the eyes of others. He needs to
see that playful light that flickers behind the pupil and makes
the eye, above all organs, eloquent, fierce, audacious, threatening, or dolorous, and equally capable of spewing forth tongues
of flame and barbs of ice.

Reminiscence of the Blind Beggar

Why the image of the blind beggar took form once again, forty
years after it had vanished, I will never know. Perhaps it was
called forth upon my reading those lines in Milton in which
the recently blinded Samson paints the terror of his sightless
state as "worse than chains,/Dungeon, or beggary, or decrepit
age!," verses whose hypnotic effect conjured the image. For
that man lived his days sunk into the triple plight of blindness,

beggary, and old age. Bitter was his lot; echoing the lamentation
of Samson, he might have claimed a status lower than that of
the vilest worm, for

> They creep, yet see; I dark in light expos'd
> To daily fraud, contempt, abuse and wrong . . .

Or else, as is more likely, the image of the blind beggar
surfaced of its own, like the cadaver of a drowned man borne
to shore by the tide of memory. For this, and nothing more, is
what memories are: corpses once consigned to the bottom of
an ocean, whence they were not to stir. And yet they rock,
slowly they rock, swayed by the ebb and flow of the green
waters, until at last they are detached from the sandy bottom
and made to drift, and cast ashore by the same pervasive movement, deceptively random, which is the natural rhythm of
remembrance.

He came every night, guided by no one, preceding each step
by that circular movement of the cane with which blind men
seem to oar across their darkness. No need to look at his hands
to know that his youth, and much of his adult age, had been
spent in the open fields, tilling the land. It was enough to look
at his cane: a veritable peasant's staff, rustic, knotty and un-
varnished, ending by way of handle in a three-armed cross, like
the Egyptian tau upon which Saint Philip endured martyrdom.

Despite his assiduous attendance, his origin, past life, and
habits were unknown to the residents—a remarkable una-
wareness in a neighborhood where everyone looked into everyone else's affairs with that sort of peering intrusion, not always
benevolent, that a social scientist may rank today a feature of
"communal life," and that wistfully we ascribe to a style of life

that is no longer possible for us. The truth remains: no one knew a thing about the old man. Sometimes, one of the women coming back from church, and still suffused by sentiments of Christian charity, would spot the beggar walking to his customary begging site in front of the store and would spontaneously offer her help in conducting him. The old man would accept this guidance, but replied to the questions ordinarily put to him in such a way as to show that his mind was not in tune with his interlocutor's. As a child, I walked by the side of these officious conductors, and I am witness to their frustration in attempting to converse with the old beggar.

For instance, asked whether anyone was to pick him up in the evening, past begging time, he would retort, "Is it after ten o'clock?" This answer could be thought of as having a logical connection with the matter of his care and assistance late at night. The questioner, therefore, could persist in trying to find out the old man's dispositions for the evening, and press him for a clear answer. A favorite second reply, also formulated in the interrogative mode, was, "Are there cows, or bulls, around here?" At this point the disconcerted questioner usually realized that the set of preconditions requisite for spoken intercourse was missing. Often, the conversation ended here.

On occasion, however, an ill-informed or naturally persevering questioner would not abandon cause. That cows or bulls should be invoked as a possible eventuality in the city streets made no sense at all. That this answer should have come up by way of reply to voiced curiosity over the old man's nightly shelter was simply absurd. And yet an overly optimistic interlocutor could find that this reply was not lacking in propriety and logic. Ten or fifteen years before, those city streets had been empty fields; perhaps in the past it had been legitimate to worry about the danger of loose cattle in the area. The city had grown fast, and an old blind man could lose track of time as easily and as utterly as of surroundings. Perhaps the old man simply needed reassurance before proceeding. By this train of subtle reasoning, a persistent questioner could conclude that the blind man was in the mood for conversation. Accordingly, after a moment's hesitation, just the time needed to go through this absolving chain of inference, a new question would be posed to the old man: where did he live, who took care of him, and the like. Virtually always, since his replies were stereotyped, the answer was, "I once danced with the First Lady." No more was needed to discourage the questioner, who hurried his pace, at times even abandoning the blind man in a street crossing.

To dismiss this strange behavior as simple madness would be unperceptive. Madness is never simple, but in this case it took on a remarkable quality, namely that it was lunacy subordinate to interaction with others, and proportional to external stimulus. The blind man's answers seemed to become progressively wilder, more nonsensical, as more questions were put to him, and as more efforts were made to engage him in conversation. Left to himself, he might have remained in an indifferent state of madness, like a plummet pointed dead center toward Bedlam; made to converse, the plummet became an activated pendulum, swinging with each exchange, and giving sanity an ever wider berth with each swing. Of all forms of madness I have come across since, this alone was not self-generated.

It is firmly set in the natural history of mental discomfitures that the deranged impulse is to come from within. Witnesses suffer it, may perhaps deflect it, but never initiate it. Yet for the blind beggar insanity was like a swing on which he sat, rocking gently, and waiting for a push. We were that baneful boost; it fell to us to increase the momentum of his malady, which was activated or worsened only from outside. I know full well that the learned will scoff at this description, and will object that an illness of this nature is yet to be reported in their ponderous archives. But I say that if such example has not yet been entered, their taxonomy is incomplete. Nor do I have the slightest doubt that the experts would agree with me had they observed, as I daily saw, the reiterative motions of the patient. Arrived at his post, the old man rocked his torso for hours, to and fro, ceaselessly, with the monotonous regularity of a met-ronome, while he sang a succession of ballads, airs of his land, all croaked rather than sung, with a doleful throaty voice that made his entire repertoire sound exactly like one and the same song, punctuated by the same tempo—the pristine rhythm, we may suppose, of his undisturbed madness.

I see him clearly, with my mind's eye, in his habitual posture. He rocks his torso back and forth, standing with his lower back leaning against the front wall of the store, three or four steps from the threshold, arms crossed, fists closed, and the heel of the hands pressed against the upper chest: the same gesture that the deaf-mute use, I am told, to signify love. This stance seems, on but slight reflection, the wrong one for my old blind man to have congealed in, during four long decades, at the bottom of my memory. For the archetypal posture of the blind is precisely the opposite of his customary stance: the arms of the blind are extended, to grope with the hands into the dark, impenetrable, and invisible surroundings. It is thus that a line of Milton that says "this dark, wide world" fails to evoke any

particular resonance in most readers but is immediately recognized by Borges, a blind man himself, as the typical production
of a blind poet. This is because, to the blind, the world is both
oppressively dark *and* enormously wide, painfully wide, much
wider than the reach of the hands, which have taken the place
of sight as tools for exploring the universe.

The songs that the old man croaked, always rocking back
and forth, were songs befitting his wretched condition. Never
the latest love lamentations, or the sugary and sensuous vulgarity
blared by the radio. Instead, he sang austere accounts of rivalries,
of widowhood, of labor strife: old songs that may have been
popular once, but had long disappeared from popular memory,
and I suspect for good reason. I could not tell if musical merit
could be attached to any; whatever music there was in them
ceased to be in passing through the old man's larynx, that
shredder of melodies, that implacable triturator of harmonies.
But if his musical gift was unimpressive, it was otherwise for
the extent of his repertoire.

Illiterate as he was, he had committed to memory an endless
succession of ballads peopled by images of women dressed in
black, of homeless children abandoned by starving mothers, of
workers exhorting one another as they faced the bosses' cronies.
I have since learned that he was not unique in this respect.
There is an ancient tradition of rude bards who discipline themselves to remember tales and ballads. Such were the Gallic Druids
who astounded Caesar by the number of unwritten verses they
could remember, or the priests of Heliopolis who caused the
admiration of Herodotus. And even as late as the nineteenth
century, says Grote, the towns of Greece were crisscrossed by
perambulating rhapsodists, all of them blind, whose job it was

to repeat, to perpetuate, and to spread, but never to increase, an enormous mass of popular songs and ballads. It is a trite convention to compare a blind rhapsodist to Homer, if there ever was such a man. I will skip the comparison: the chasm seems too wide between the man—or men—who uttered the epic of epics for all time to come, and the old man who begged near the door of my neighborhood drugstore. However altered his image may have surfaced out of the sea of memory, the seaweed that clings to his brow does not resemble the crown of laurel. And he remains a toothless, gaunt, squalid being, rapped by life on the head with such strong blows as to leave him an idiotic wreck, bobbing to and fro, like flotsam on shaken waters.

The neighborhood changed. The number of kind ladies given to weekly spasms of Christian charity remained constant, but the number of jobless adolescent males increased disproportionately. Or so it seemed from the gathered groups of young ruffians at every corner. At every street corner, that is, from which women could be ogled, and dice rolled, and bottles passed from hand to hand in a circle. It was inevitable that this coterie of young toughs, growing heady as the contents of their bottles dwindled, would not remain indifferent to the ever-rocking minstrel. On that baneful day they began by mocking among themselves those strange narratives of firing squads, of disheveled mothers holding infants to their dry breasts, and of workers martyred at the hands of infamous strikebreakers. The rocking motion of the old man was then made the target of their jokes: one, then two, then a whole row of young punks stood side by side with the beggar, imitating his repetitive movements, rocking in unison with him, arms crossed against the upper chest. At last the raspy voice was the butt of the satire, and great mirth was elicited by the improvised imitations of the belchlike, syncopated sounds of the beggar.

No one could tell if the semi-demented old man was conscious of being mocked. But it was plain that the commotion and laughter disturbed him. And the observant might have judged the magnitude of his trouble by one outward sign: he lost his rhythm; that deepest emanation of his undisturbed inner being came undone. The rocking, for years stereotyped in an unvarying tempo, became irregular and discontinuous, as if chopped to pieces by those young intruders who lowered him gradually into a pit of anxiety. Next, his ballads became mixed up, the thread of the narrative so hopelessly entangled that the account that began with the abandoned orphan was continued with the designs of vengeance of the prisoner, and concluded with the tale of workers' solidarity. At last, the pitiable old man made an abrupt halt in his singing. His lusterless corneas revolved nervously in their orbits, as if trying to relearn in one second the long-lost habit of their searching motions. The old man asked, in a loud voice, whether it was past ten o'clock, whether there were any bulls in the area, and then peremptorily declared that he had once danced with the First Lady.

Each one of these utterances fueled the collective mirth and provoked clownish repartees from his taunters. Emboldened by their success in confusing the old man, they passed from parodying his gestures to touching him, startling him, tapping him. This one would hold him by one hand while grotesquely simulating the steps of a dance; that one would nudge him in the ribs with the forehead while imitating the lowing of cattle. Suddenly the callused fist closed itself on the wooden cane that rested against the wall, and the beggar advanced, reeling about and discharging furious blows with his cane, violent slashes that whistled in the air.

There was a generalized scampering for cover and cries of alarm. There were wailing expressions of dismay from the kind ladies of intermittent Christian charity, who could not believe their eyes, that there should be young men so heartless as to make an old blind beggar the object of their pranks. However, the old man was transformed. He was, at that moment, far from defenseless. He swung his cane in circular movements and turned about abruptly, thrusting now from left to right, now from right to left; and then, advancing with his cane held high, like a drunken landsknecht with a two-handed sword, discharged mighty blows, swinging his arm up and down. The risk of bodily harm held the spectators at a prudent distance, but only added spice to the boys' game. The amusement now consisted of braving danger in various ways: to wait for the thrust to spend its energy, then to come from behind the old man, and to scream at the top of one's lungs, "It is past ten o'clock!"; and, as soon as the blind man would charge against the unseen offender, to come at him again from an unsuspected angle, imitating the lowing of cattle; and so on, while the enraged old man went forth shouting obscenities, staggering along, reeling about himself, and discharging blows with his cane.

The image of the old, blind beggar has resurfaced in this setting, last of my memories of his likeness. The colored neon lights of the drugstore's street signs went on and off intermittently, and fell upon the sweaty countenance of the toothless old man. And his face, with its dull whitish corneas, became red, yellow, blue, and green, and again red, yellow, blue, and green at each gyration, while he held the rustic cane above his head. Just so Moses must have looked, brightened with lights from heaven when he elevated the serpent and held it high at the tip of his staff. But in the context of ordinary experience, my blind old man's dim understanding was as hopelessly remote from the spirit of the prophet as the streets on which he suffered lay distant from the road to salvation.

His staff did come down. It landed—what dark forces directed it?—on the skull of an inadvertent passerby. Not one of his tormentors, but an altogether unconcerned adolescent girl on an errand, as she came out of the drugstore. There was a terrible sound, such as is aptly compared to the cracking of a hollow earthenware pot, and a limp body collapsing, while rivulets of blood meandered over the pale face. And only then did the able-bodied men who had stood watching the previous scenes with amusement throw themselves over the beggar to subdue him. Amid the screams of the terrified kind ladies, the whey-faced victim was lifted by the armpits and dragged toward the lee of the drugstore's front wall, there to wait for the ambulance.

There is no more to add. The whereabouts of the beggar remained, after that fateful night, as mysterious as had been his origin and manner of life. The question is whether the entire substance of this episode, this vulgar episode, may be compressed into a few visual images that are then submerged into the depths of memory, or whether a hidden meaning, "unseen" but discoverable, exists behind the images. I make no apologies for having ardently wished to believe, all these years, that the episode was explainable; that a blind, old, demented beggar ridiculed and taunted by irresponsible youths was an occurrence of only apparent senselessness; that the old man's idiotic wrath falling upon the head of an innocent child was a happening that seemed absurd only after superficial examination; but that the entire scene could be fitted into a logical pattern, a necessary and orderly arrangement, if only the key to this disturbing puzzle were looked for earnestly enough.

I make no apologies, I say, for having wished to avert "the mind's eye" from protracted contemplation of the absurd. For I have discovered that seeing is among the most difficult tasks that confront us. How to cope with the multifarious spectacle of the world is a delicate art that few master. The hysteric patient who finds reality too painful to bear resorts to a "conversion reaction" that constricts the field of vision, or blots it out entirely, without organic impairment of the eyes. The more sanguine can take in sights uplifting or degrading, the hurtful with the soothing, as mere animal sense data to be stored unexamined—and let the images resurface when they will. Mystics denounce vision, and all sense perceptions, as dark veils woven of carnal solicitations that impede the view of a transcendent reality hidden behind the outward face of things. They speak of two different "eyesights," the one bodily, the other angelical; that one collecting purely animal, sensual impressions; and this one destined to gather the highest spiritual illuminations.

The middle course, therefore, would require us to see and not to see, to admit the images that impress the retina and discard them straight away in order to attain a superior insight. But no one will teach us how to achieve this difficult feat. Mystics least of all, who omit description of technique and speak in parables. Some thought of God as one-eyed: the spiritual eye open, the carnal one shut. In the iconography of some ancient devotional works, God the Father and Jesus his Son appear represented as monocular. Tauler, a medieval theologian, enjoined his flock to concentrate on spiritual vision by disdaining corporeal sight, "just as the marksman shuts one eye to sharpen the vision of the other." What does this mean? We are not told. Perhaps nothing at all. Perhaps this is simply an image to be stored, under a thousand others, in the green waters of memory—to resurface when it will.

TASTE

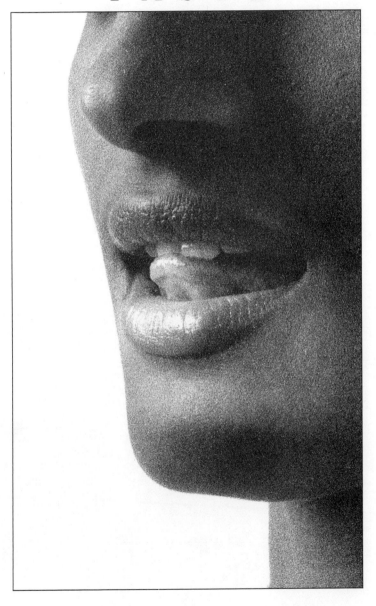

Reminiscences of a Hot-Pepper Eater

WHAT IT IS that first compelled Mexicans to relish murderous hot peppers, like dainties, may be discussed without profit until the end of time. It was not an epicurean tendency. The first man who made a habit of eating them could not have been in a state of mind to agree with Epicurus that "voluptuousness is the supreme good." No; to decide that these acrid, flaming, scorching plants are edible, one must be in some extreme state, where all thoughts are for self-preservation, or for self-denial. A balanced or sedate disposition never would have dreamed of creating such cookery.

On the other hand, the nature of these sauces comported with the spirit and temper of my father. He was a child of disordered times, and had grown to be a man of unusual propensities. The fiery assaults on his tongue he had learned to withstand, then to like. As many of his countrymen still do, he taught himself, by assiduous and gradual exposure, a perfect tolerance to concoctions that, if accidentally spilled, would have bored into the table and straight through the planks of the floor.

I did not know the details of this inurement. But I learned that for some time he had subsisted out of a diet made principally of those scorchers. My father had served in the ranks of one of the many self-appointed "generals" of the Mexican Revolution in the early part of this century. He spoke of being awakened at daybreak by the stirring sound of the trumpet; of planting dynamite charges under train tracks, to derail the enemy convoys; and of remaining still for hours in the company of his confederates, "lying on the ground like lizards," when setting

up ambushes under a scorching sun. These narratives touched
my youthful imagination. They told of a legion of heroic men
who fought on arid, hostile lands, men who marched in single
file over rough trails crossed by rattlesnakes while buzzards
circled in the air above them, men who endured privations
untold, carrying obsolete Belgian-made rifles, amidst agave plants
that barely managed to suck traces of humidity from the very
rocks in which they grew. When the men encamped on some
desolate hill, the sole means of relieving their parched tongues
was to open the pulpy disk of some cactus, defended by for-
bidding, enormous thorns. When heatstroke threatened, they
found no foliage to shade them, only the thin, tall silhouette of
the "candle" cactus, whose most merciful concession is to grow
sometimes in parallel rows, like the pickets of a fence.

According to my father, so profound was the impress of this
pitiless landscape that men's characters were shaped in its image
and semblance. Those who survived became petrous and insen-
sitive, like the land. They needed no comfort, and shunned
softness in men or in things. Only thus was it conceivable that
at night, when their bivouacs went up, they should still crave
the fiery condiment and feel no need to rinse the burning
sensation with the scant water from some brackish pond. They
were indeed a hardy race, pugnacious and heroic, and worthy
of Xenophon's Anabasis. Tempered by fire, like swordblades, they
naturally came to crave fire for their sustenance.

Or so my father said. When his stories of the taking of a
town came up at dinnertime, my mother evinced a discreet but
unmistakable indifference. Through the distant crackling of gun-
fire, and the anecdotal references to "my general Orozco," she
carried on with her housewifely duties, more attentive to the

state of the silverware than to the destinies of the nation or the fortunes of war. Once, in an aside carefully calculated for my ears only, she replied to my curiosity with a chilling comment: "You know how your father is. You must not believe everything he says." He must have sensed the lack of accord with his audience. His storytelling never amounted to more than quick and stumped sketches, never giving us the complete sum and substance of his participation in the grandiose saga.

Interest on my part was not wanting; a young boy is naturally captivated by tales of adventure. But it must be owned that the degree of my enthusiasm fell short of his expectations. By that perverse, arcane system of compensations that gives the pious man a miscreant for a son, or bequeaths morose offspring to the sharp-witted, my father had managed to sire a poltroon. The man of action had, as his only son, a retiring lad who would fain sit reading the thick volumes of the Doré collection and gazing at the wonderful engravings sooner than feel the need to emulate, in actual deed, the feats of heroism therein portrayed. After some hesitation, my father would voluntarily withdraw from the narratives of military prowess to the mundane concerns of settled life, and the dinner continued.

Those were postrevolutionary days, when dashing hardihood had become either redundant or unseemly. The skills most in demand were of the sort my father was wanting. The world had grown complex. A man sustained chiefly by dreams of glory, hope for sudden riches, and trust in feats of audacity no longer commanded the same attention as before. One evening he grew somber, dipped one more time into the plate containing the pungent, acrid spices that he loved so much, and, noticing that I had carefully avoided partaking of the devilish condiment, sprinkled a generous dose on my dish. A few minutes later, my tastebuds contacted the fiercest, meanest seeds in the botanical world. It was as if flames had hit every portion of my oral mucosa, or as if, by freak and monstrous accident, I had swallowed vitriol. Unable to speak, I held my neck with my left hand, while with my right I made fanning motions, as if trying to extinguish the fire inside my mouth, through which instinctively I protruded an acutely suffering, trembling tongue. The spectacle of my tearing eyes and flushed face moved my mother to give me leave to quit the table. My father said, impatiently, "What is the matter with this fellow? Is he not a Mexican?" and seemed to wish to stop me. "Leave him alone," rejoined my mother. "You can see that he is just a boy." And I quickly ran to the bathroon, for rinsings, washings, undisturbed salivation, and indulgent self-commiseration.

To his credit, this was the only time that he attempted to make a he-man out of a spineless, softish boy. He was always respectful of my mother's wishes. And then he had plenty of other things to worry about—most of all his own self, in deep, schismatic disaccord with the temper of the times.

Nothing is more grievously poignant than the spectacle of a man at odds with his circumstance. This was his plight. He was fixed in time, improvident and unrealistic. Others knew that our society had suffered a violent wrenching and dislocation, when only luck availed, as in an earthquake; when only prompt and rash action counted, as in a conflagration; and when only faith and resilience saved, as in a shipwreck. But those times were past. The tumultuous and disordered life was followed by a relative calm; and the qualities that had helped in the former, hindered in the latter. Now that it was imperative to cultivate the solid and tangible benefits, my father still clung to a thousand apparitions.

One, in particular, recurred with insistence. While on patrol, he said, he had wandered into enemy territory and narrowly escaped being made a prisoner. During his perilous flight he descended into a deep ravine and discovered the entrance to an abandoned mine that he knew existed in the area. He lowered himself into the tunnels and walked the underground passageways for as long as he suspected that the *federales*, enemy troops, were still aboveground. He was never the same after he emerged again to the dazzle of sunlight. In that cavernous hideout he had seen the promise of riches beyond belief. The entrails of the earth were made of silver tissues, and he had seen them, touched them, trodden upon their very woof. The darkness of those galleries yielded to the glimmer of precious streaks embedded in the rock. Experience, which in most men successfully dissipates illusion, never could perform its spiteful work in my father after he had seen the mine. Thereafter he lived under the potent spell cast by the underground passageways.

He returned there after the troubles were over. He reinspected the galleries, and again palpated the tantalizing raw wealth that awaited him there, "for the taking." His delusions were only strengthened. If it is true that mind is the sole depository of happiness, never was my father so happy as in those days, with his mind buoyed in the elation of anticipated opulence. His present insecurity lost its terror; his life became invested with new meaning; hope compelled all his worries into perpetual banishment. He knew the area very well, for the mine was in his native state. All the local people knew of its existence but, simple rural characters that they were, the prospects of

exploiting the buried riches fell beyond the narrow circum-
scription of their aspirations and abilities. He questioned the
local inhabitants on the history of the mine. Their stories, em-
bellished by time and imagination, made in him a profound
impression.

The first owner had been a Spaniard, in colonial times. The
oral tradition maintained that his likeness was represented in a
mediocre oil painting at the town church. He appeared as a
kneeling figure dressed in ancient habiliments of black brocade,
at the foot of a levitating Saint Agatha. A bluish shade over his
clean-shaven chin and mandible premonished a dense black
beard over his olive skin. But this devout worshiper frozen in
mystical transport while contemplating the heavenly portent,
had been in reality a remorseless slave driver. He forced the
miners to toil without rest, crawling on all fours all the time,
in the most inhumane conditions, until the stony sides of the
mountain were split wide open. He vowed to decorate with
jewels the mantle of Our Lady of Pilar, in his native town, if
he found the deposit of silver that obsessed him. His wish was
granted, and as riches upon riches were lavished on him, the
velvet cloak of the Immaculate Mother of God in some obscure
Spanish town became dotted with rubies, sapphires, emeralds,
and hyacinths.

Silver continued to pour out, thanks to the ceaseless hacking
and shoveling of hundreds of indigent Indians with harnesses
around their waists, and chains between their legs, whom the
Spaniard fustigated mercilessly while a cold glimmer of cruelty
passed through his pitch-black eyes. The Spanish Virgin of his
hometown now donned a massive imperial crown, and a large

aureole with rays of the purest gold, but huge loads of the mine's silver were still forthcoming.

At last, after close to twenty years, the rapacious Spaniard was found stabbed, a corpse half-devoured by vultures in some craggy place. Whether a rival had murdered him to satisfy ambitious designs or whether a poor underground drudge, maddened by his awful oppression, had seen fit to take justice in his own hands was never known. But it was a widely held belief among the villagers all around the mine that the Spaniard's last wish and testament provided for the complete decoration of his hometown church with silver. None of the humble villagers could name the town of his birthplace, but none doubted that there existed, somewhere in the Iberian peninsula, a church with gorgeous altars of sterling, and enormous silver caskets, and crosses, and crucifixes of the same metal; a church where even the pillars were encrusted with silver ornaments, and the paintings held by silver frames, and the floor tiles interlaid with silver ingots; a church where huge silver saints flanked the central image of Our Lady of Pilar, whose shoulders had been covered by a mantle studded with precious stones—the stones purchased with the silver of the Mexican mine.

The last owner had been a corpulent Northerner. Whether German or Scandinavian, the old-timers did not always agree. "Gringos look all alike, you know, like the Chinese" was the comment of an old man. All agreed, however, that the man spoke an unintelligible language, and peered at the world through sky-blue eyes. His pink-reddish complexion could turn beet-red when in a temper, and his flaxen hair grew down into muttonchops on both sides of his head. Although not as fiercely malevolent as the Spaniard, he was equally ambitious. With indefatigable drive, and using updated equipment, in a short time he pulled out tons of the inexhaustible metal. But the climate of the region suited him badly, and he fell ill. At length he decided that he would spend the rest of his days, which he guessed were growing scant, in his homeland.

The crews of foreign technicians absconded; the cranes were disassembled; and the equipment and machines, the purpose of many of them a mystery, were put in crates and shipped off. The corpulent Norseman, immensely rich, went back to his country, whether in Bavaria or in Denmark the people could not say. But all of them were ready to swear, on the evidence of a postcard that a foreman later received, that he had ended his days in a sumptuous castle with dozens of rooms in the midst of a thickly wooded, noble forest; and that he spent his time tended by black-suited butlers, blue-eyed like himself, who ceremoniously served him tea from silver pots carried on silver trays, which they daily buffed to a perfect shine.

These were the stories that my father repeated, growing animated and flushed as he dipped the wooden spoon into the steaming-hot pepper sauce.

"Do you really believe that the Spaniard tiled the whole floor of his church with silver?"

"Not the *whole* floor. The priest of my hometown has been to Spain. He says there is a line of ingots going from the portico to the center of the altar, along the central aisle. You know, that madman wished to pave the whole route from his house to the church's altar with silver, just so his daughter could walk on silver all the way to the church when she got married. I think he could have done it, if the town's authorities had given him permission to execute that crazy idea."

"And the stories about the gringo, do you believe those, too?"

"He was not a gringo, he was Swedish. And what is wrong with those stories? Let me tell you, when the new agrarian laws were proclaimed, I was with my general Orozco, and we confiscated a huge hacienda up in the mountains, the property of an English couple. Do you believe that they received us in formal dress? In the middle of the sierra, when the revolution was raging all around them, and where only wildcats and raccoons called at their door, they had kept up their custom of dressing formally for dinner. The man was in black tuxedo and tie, the woman in long dress. You can never understand those people, no matter how hard you try! No, I am not at all surprised at the stories that are said about the Swedish."

With this kind of unswerving conviction my father deflected objections to his plans. Never mind that he had not the foggiest inkling of the technical aspects that govern the mining process, or the appropriate means to contact those who did: no true obstacle ever stood in the way of genuine enthusiasm. To suggest that a productive mine is not suddenly abandoned without a reason, or that its neglect foreboded ill, was to provoke his most impassioned addresses. Timorousness, he said, was the national disgrace. So long as this self-effacing attitude prevailed, Mexicans were condemned to stand aside while foreigners exploited the land, dug out the subsoil, fished in our seas, and took away all the riches that were rightfully ours. Was it not time to take our destiny in our own hands? Was this not, in fact, the reason why the revolution had been fought? Unless, of course, a lackey mentality was so deeply imprinted in you that you did not have the nerve for grand and lofty enterprise. In that case, you might as well be content with the scraps that you could eke out day by day, and let the foreigners keep helping themselves to the bounteous treasures of our native soil.

Visionary zeal wedded to nationalistic appeal formed a powerful combination. The sincerity of the haranguer was moving, and it was not long before he had made adepts. The mining business is complex, and he needed managers, administrators, people of polish and education who could move with ease among capitalists, investors, and mining engineers. The trouble was, my father was impractical, unrealistic, and fantasy-prone. He naturally gravitated toward a motley crowd than which no more exotic and colorful can be found in the most outlandish creations of farcical writers. One such was Mrs. X., nicknamed "the Duchess," a withered South American dame with blue-painted grotesque shadows around the rims of her eyes who used preposterously long cigarette holders with gilded tips and wore flashy turbans with plumed adornments, like a Hindu maharani's, and elbow-length gloves that she studiously protected from being soiled when visiting our house. The first time she came to visit, asking for my father by his first name and evincing undisguised repugnance at the modesty of our lodgings, my mother saluted her with glances scarcely less lethal than the Borgias' potions.

There was also Mr. J., a mysterious man of uncertain origin with bushy eyebrows and gold-rimmed spectacles. He had lived in Cuba and had acquired, there perhaps, a taste for white suits and white shoes, as well as Panama hats. This attire was complemented by a red bandanna tied around his neck, and a silky handkerchief to match, protruding from his jacket chest pocket. He was obviously a man of not negligible worldly experience, but it had been, I am afraid, chiefly of a sleazy sort; in a word, not the most desirable associate for an inexperienced business-man. Mr. J.'s tendency to appear at our house during my father's absence, and his legerdemain in passing his hirsute fingers over my young mother's arms and shoulders, educed glances from her almost as poisonous as those she directed to my father's female business associate.

Where did all these strange people come from? By what uncanny influences did they converge at that time, responding to the appeal of my father's delusions? When, many years later, I posed these questions to my mother, she replied matter-of-factly, "They came from the deep, as sharks do when they sense that there is blood to be had." In those days, however, all was conviviality among presumptive predators and preys. There were dinners at which my father's lingual fortitude was the celebrated centerpiece of the conversation; loud exclamations and laughter when others dared to taste his infernal sauces; sessions at which spiritous imbibing disfurnished my father of his minuscule al-lotment of common sense and ended with his signing, in a foggy stupor, such documents as might have required sober canvassing and fastidious deliberation. This unlikely team generated more action than seemed possible. The suggestion of material profit evidently makes the wildest plans seem plausible. A mining company was founded; stock was sold; certificates were printed; and an office with all the trappings of respectability was rented in a plush building, downtown. Then came the day to visit the mine for the official inauguration.

My parents and I set out for the roughest regions of my

father's native state. We alighted at his family homestead, late
in the evening. For the welcoming meal, the next day, a special
hot sauce was prepared. A servant girl had been out to pick a
variety of hot pepper that grew in the environs and passed for
the most unbearably hot species that the land could support.
In the kitchen, the women had ground an assortment of peppers
in their *molcajetes*, mortarlike stone receptacles in which Indian
women manually grind seasonings with a fist-sized stone for a
pestle. The occasion was a memorable one. My father's fire-
craving nature was known, and, by way of challenge, an explosive
mixture of the most acrid, stinging, scorching grains and plant
juices had been prepared. The cooks were careful to avoid skin
contact, lest blisters be raised. The mere effluvia stung one's
eyes; I suspect metallic spoons would have melted if they had
been left to soak in the mixture. Amidst the giggling and grinning
of the women, and the stares of the men, who shook their heads
in disbelief at his prowess, my father finished the smoking
concoction without flinching, and protested that it "had no
bite." Replied a vivacious young Indian woman, to the merriment of the assembly, "Tomorrow, sir, I shall go hunting for a
live rattler. Palates such as yours will reckon no bite in anything
less malignant."

I was quite impressed. In those days my father cut a dashing
figure: tall, trim, with handsome Spanish features. He had come
to the heart of an acrid land, and had exceeded the most daring
feats of this fire-eating race. Quickened by the jollity of the
group, I dared to taste a tiny sample at the tip of my table
knife. The fiery blast sent me whimpering into my mother's
arms.

We then trekked across inhospitable hills and valleys, along narrow, pebbly trails. Had I been of an age to reason maturely, I would have wondered how the mined products were going to be transported. I do not know if anyone did. At length we made it to the entrance of the old mine, a yawning black hole from which the wild brush had just been cleared. A wooden sign had been affixed on two poles, with the name of the mine, Esperanza, in red paint. *Esperanza* means "hope," and is also a woman's name. The appellations of mines, like those of hurricanes, were often feminine. This partiality for femininity did not preclude the foreman from barring my mother's entry to the mine. It was thought to be bad luck, he said, if a woman approached the labyrinthine galleries before the exploitation had begun. She stayed in the sun while an all-male party, armed with flashlights, made for the netherworld. I was of their number.

I don't remember how long we walked in the dimly lit galleries before we encountered water covering the ground. As an ingratiating gesture toward my father, the foreman, who walked in front, took me in his arms, and we continued our progress until the water reached up to his waist. Here the gallery ended in a cul-de-sac. The men shone their flashlights on the rocky walls, revealing a wonderful spectacle. The rough, jagged black stone seemed adorned with glistening sequins and silver threads. In places, it was as if a shiny white powder had been sprinkled over the irregular surface of a stony meteorite; in other places, as if a silvery venation had been disposed in capricious arabesques throughout the gallery. We were spellbound. We had entered a subterranean Alhambra, whose magnificent walls were ornamented on every square inch with silvery patterns of ineffable beauty. The magical effect was heightened by

the deep silence that prevailed in the depths of the earth. And
the whole shone, scintillated, sparkled under the unsteady beams
of the hand-held flashlights. The men fell silent for a few minutes
and then made fervid comments in which a word which I heard
for the first time, *la veta*, "the ore," was pronounced with all
the wistful intensity of a religious invocation. We returned to
the sunlight.

The foreman arrayed the miners, some thirty men, in frontal
formation before the mine entrance, carrying their working
tools, like men-at-arms with weapons, for the long, rectangular
group photograph that was to hang at the company's head-
quarters in Mexico City. This raggedy band of peasants, momentarily snatched to the glebe, held in their hands a few picks,
shovels, and land-tilling instruments: no mining had taken place
in the region for close to fifty years. I recollect no machinery,
no hydraulic gear, no electricity-driven carts or elevators such
as one expects to see in mines. Of the company's executive
cadre, only my father and two clerks, who were also his relatives,
attended the inauguration. Mr. J. had to stay behind for an
interview with potential investors, who at this very moment
were engulfed in a double cloud of Havana cigar smoke and
suave rhetoric. Mrs. Z., alias "the Duchess," superintended the
last details of the central office's interior decoration. No matter.
We posed, just the same, for the group photograph; I, my hand
held by the foreman, in the center of the picture.

From the calculating viewpoint of, say, a foreign investor,
we probably looked more like one of the unruly bands of peasants
that followed Zapata, or some other revolutionary chieftain (and
with good reason, since some of the participants had, in fact,
served under Zapata), than a disciplined group of well-equipped

miners about to realize a great profit for the controlling interests of finance. But from my father's perspective we were both the symbol of his personal fortune and the vindicators of the national honor. No more would foreign exploiters steal the riches that were ours. From now on, through his example and his organizer's talent, the motherland would open her bounty to her sons. Toil and harshness still lay ahead, but in the end a rich reward awaited, as much for his individual solace as for the admiration of the world. A dreamer: impractical, unrealistic, and misguided. That is how he was.

Before leaving the place we stopped by the church. A priest had not been summoned to bless the mine. Despite his anti-clerical prejudice, my father was persuaded at the last moment that it was a wise move to impress the miners with the idea that our enterprise was not one to reject the good auspices of the nation's secular religion. I stayed in the sacristy while a delegation arranged with the priest for a new ceremony at which Esperanza would be officially baptized. In the sacristy, behind an espadrilled arch, stood the patinated portrait of the Spaniard, still absorbed in contemplation of Saint Agatha, who levitated to heaven in a golden mist. We left the town, and returned to the big city that same evening.

Esperanza turned out to be a *femme fatale*. Fickle and ungrateful like Mérimée's *Carmen*, insatiable and demanding like Zola's *Nana*, in man-eating propensity she exceeded them both. Nothing sufficed for her upkeep. Week after week new gifts and donations were offered her, but she was never satisfied. All that she had given out formerly—the precious cargoes that Spaniards had transported in galleons with the colors of Castile flaming atop their masts; the tons of ingots loaded by fair-haired men into ships that had sailed to embayments and passed through fjords flanked by ice-capped peaks; the mountainous heaps of metal that Americans had disinterred and then buried again underground in vaults in California or New York, to support the arts of peace and the industry of war—*all* she wanted back.

My father, who had chosen the carbine and the cartridge belt across his chest to fight an oppressive government, now put on the shining armor of illness and took up the sword of alcoholism to do battle against a bloodsucking mine. He locked himself in the bedroom and drew curtains about him. Mr. J. appeared twice, nervously brandishing notes, accounts receivable, demands for payment of miners' wages and for purchase of water-pumping equipment; Mrs. Z. once, fleetingly, only to leave us the immanent trace of her cheap cologne, and the tinkling of her earrings, and armbands, and wristbands. But all this had for my father as much relevance as if it had happened on a distant star. In the alcoholic oblivion in which he sank the word "payment" had lost its meaning; the words "legal suit" were an absurdity for him; and the talk of financial ruin sounded like meaningless noise. His mind was effectively shut up in an ethylic bubble, and there he felt safe from the disagreeable impressions that the world presumed to force upon him.

Strange to recount, while visited with these appalling calamities my father showed no appetite for food, properly so-called. In the evident state of inanition in which he lived, retired from the notice of the world and ignorant of what passed out-of-doors, he eluded the universal law of nature. He sustained himself exclusively with wine, and, incredibly, with soupy concoctions of his ever-present hot peppers. The maid, an Indian girl from his native state, still drew out every morning the many varieties of hot peppers that were kept in the pantry: ancho, piquín, jalapeño; yellow, green, black, or crimson red. To these she added the extremely pungent, many-seeded pods of the pepper that grew only in the rough hills around the mine, whence the flaming specimens were periodically shipped to our house.

My mother brought more substantive dishes to his bedroom and placed them beside the earthenware plate of hot-pepper broth. At night, the former were withdrawn untouched, the latter empty. Obviously, in his feverish state of mind, his preference turned wholly to dishes that burn, rather than gratify, the appetite. I have sometimes wondered about this characteristic of Mexican cookery. Scholars believe that the strange condiments were developed first by Aztec sacrificers, and later elaborated upon by novices of Spanish or mixed blood, who used to read accounts of transfigurations, torments, and martyrdoms in the solitude of their convents. And so I fancy that this double genealogy, with its disquieting tendencies, may have shown itself in my father as a craving for some form of sense-transcending, fire-eating ecstasy. But this is idle speculation. There were, at the time, much more pressing concerns related to his oral deviancy. A physician came to see him, and to give him injections of vitamins. "Should we do anything, doctor," said my mother, "to deter him from those awful hot peppers? They are giving him an ulcer." "My dear lady," said he, "I have never seen such an extraordinary perversion of the appetite. But there's a habit more pernicious than tongue-burning, and it is killing him. I would rather keep him away from the bottle."

The mine's revenge was not appeased. The awesome telluric

vengeance now created an immense suction force, a centripetal field that pulled everything mightily toward itself. First, the wooden props that supported the galleries; then, the sediment layers that eons of geological aging had deposited above the mine's tunnels; then, the masses of porphyritic rock; then the bones of extinct animals enmeshed in rocks and subsoil and muddy earth; then, the layer of greensward with the roots of trees and plants; and even the animals that feed on them; and the houses that rest on the earth's surface; and the men who toil, and dream, and die, and are buried in the earth. All was pulled into the maelstrom. All came spiraling down, toward the center of the rocky galleries, adorned with silvery, sparkling inlays. And then, after the great vortex had sucked in even the roots of the hot pepper plants that grew thousands of yards above the galleries, the great suction force came to be exerted upon my father's viscera, connected, as they were, to those plants by the invisible moorings of perpetual craving.

Sooner or later it had to find him. Then, one day, the overwhelming suction reached my father's stomach. He felt it coming, and tried to withstand the incommensurable whirling blast by holding on, as hard as he could, with his hands on each side of the lavatory. But the force was too great, and it attained his insides. He retched violently, curving his body toward the lavatory. His eyes turned red, and seemed to pop out. The small capillaries of his conjunctivas were intensely congested, and the veins on his temples were swollen, and yet the suction force that had originated in the mine would not cease. Then this maelstrom, this whirlwind, this turbination yanked him off his hold and sent him tumbling to the floor. He still clung desperately to the solid objects about him, and held on to both sides of the toilet with his hands, kneeling on the floor. But the suction force was too great; it pulled on his stomach, on his bowel, and on his penetralia. He retched, and strained, and vomited, until, by a terrible effort, all the liquor had been ejected, all the hot-pepper soup had been emptied; and this was followed by vomiting of blackish grumous residues; and then, finally, gushes of bright red blood. When the suctioning force abated, I found him unconscious, lying in a puddle of blood, unshaved for days, and with his pajamas soiled by vomitus and dejecta.

I was kept ignorant of the many devastations that the whirlwind caused along its path. But I was witness to some of the last crushings and uprootings wrought by the subsiding winds. Mr. J. could not be found. He was tossed violently in the air, but he was quite resourceful, and controlled the impelling force to direct him back to Cuba. There he was later spotted, sipping a martini by the beachside in his impeccable white garb. The reports were contradictory, but some maintained that Mrs. Z. was with him; others, that she had been blown off to South America. The whereabouts of my father were kept hidden, even from me. The whirlwind first threw him into a hospital, then to parts unknown. Therefore, when the lawyers and notaries appeared at our house, there was only my mother to receive the full force of the gale, already quieting down but still strong, straight on her face. It made her flush, and wring her hands, and cry, and plead for mercy. The secretaries unpacked their portable typewriters. Affidavits and depositions were drawn up, and the furniture was taken out of our house by porters who had waited outside, in a truck, for the legal proceedings of repossession to be completed.

Everything that appeared new came under suspicion of being acquired by ill-gotten gain. Thus, everything new, or apparently valuable, was repossessed. In the exercise of their function, which was to restore the balance of justice, and to compensate defrauded investors for the infringement of their rights and the loss of property through trickery and misstatement, the lawyers may have overstepped their duty. I say this because, even though the loss of cupboards and armchairs and sofas never troubled me, the sudden departure of twenty richly bound volumes entitled *El Tesoro de la Juventud* (*Youth's Treasure*), plus the six or seven volumes of the Doré collection, struck me as a trifle excessive: did requitement of the wronged investors demand that Tasso and Cervantes be tied with strings, like common criminals, and thrown at their feet for satisfaction? My mother, with visible affliction, constantly ran from lawyers to porters to me, ever reassuring me that the losses were only transitory, that she would "make it up" to me, and that the volumes would be repurchased.

They never were. In my mind's eye, I saw the books whirling in the void, falling down far, very far from me, while their pages flapped in disorder in the wind, flittingly exposing the magnificent engravings that the genius of Gustave Doré had once conceived. This was the last episode of ruin and devastation caused by a mine with the name of Esperanza. It took place belatedly, months after the whirlwinds had wrought the worst disaster, as one sees precariously supported structures tumbling down amidst the rubble some time after the earthquake.

One day, as I returned from a hike in the countryside (my mother had insisted that I join a Boy Scout group, as an expedient to keep me away from an unsettled home environment),

I was informed, somewhat gently, that my father had died. As he felt death approaching, he had requested that he be transported to his native state. We had to hurry to get there before the burial. A relative who had been a clerk in the ill-fated company offered to drive us there. I saw again, for the last time, the agave plants, like upright feather dusters, opening their prickly leaves to collect the morning dew; the silhouettes of thorny cactuses, detaching themselves from the dusty air with the neatness of heraldic symbols; and the bleak, bone-dry hills, gradually growing shadowless under a perpendicular sun.

The funeral preparation was a fitting ceremonial in this immense and hopeless landscape. I was shown into the room where the open-lidded coffin was kept. Black-shawled women sat in a row of chairs flanking the walls. The coffin seemed enormous to me: placed on a high support provided by the funeral director, its upper border exceeded my stature. The crowded wreaths and bouquets of white flowers—"dead man's flower," or *flor de muerto*—imparted a musty, enervating odor to the room. Close to the door there was a small table displaying a coffee pot, liquor, and victuals, as was the custom. A woman was kneeling in front of the coffin, her black shawl drawn over her head and shoulders, and holding a rosary in her hands. She voiced a litany with her raspy voice, and to each of her invocations the rest of the women replied in a monotonous chorus, "Pray for him." I heard:

> Holy Mary,
> > Pray for him;
> Mother of God,
> > Pray for him;

> Purest Mother,
>> Pray for him;
> Immaculate Mother,
>> Pray for him.

Dolorous Mother; Rose of Heaven; Crown of the Empyrean; Support of the Fallen; Road of Salvation; Mother of Christ . . . by how many names was the celestial queen invoked and her magnanimous intercession implored? There was a moment of hesitation as I entered the room. The whispers of the women, most of whom had never seen me, spread the news that I was the son of the deceased. There followed a whispered discussion on the propriety of having me there, given my short years, and on the advisability of letting me see the mortal remains of my father. Before a consensus was reached, the man who had driven us to the town held me from behind and hoisted me to a grown man's height, from which I could look down on the open coffin window at my father's countenance.

The sight engraved itself indelibly upon my mind. It would have been untrue to say that he "rested" there. The custom of embalming cadavers is alien to the country, and my father had been deposed in precisely the attitude in which death had surprised him. His eyebrows were partly lifted and drawn together. His eyelids had not been completely closed. His brow was coursed by furrows running vertically. A yellowish tinge of the skin confirmed the diagnostic ability of our family physician: the liver, not the stomach, had been first to yield to the reiterated insult of unwholesome ingestions.

What intrigued me the most was the singular expression that resulted from the vertical furrows in the forehead, and the consequent wrinkling and incurving of the median halves of the eyebrows, like two horizontally traced question marks. This image has never left me. Yet it would not be true to say that it haunted me: never did I view it with terror, or in nightmares, or with a troubled and uneasy heart. Rather, it became for me a source of intense and unremitting curiosity: a gnawing yearning to decipher the meaning of that facial expression. Had his last moments been painful? Was that the face of a man in pain? Yet, physical pain alone could not account for a countenance in which the expressive components of bewilderment, surprise, expectation, annoyance, apprehension, and dismay seemed to blend in an intriguing mixture. Many a time I tried, alone, in front of a mirror, like an actor of mime rehearsing his routine, to reproduce exactly my father's last facial expression. I thus tried to reconstruct by a retrospective method, as it were, the possible meaning behind the visage: "Given a man with this facial expression, what thoughts, what feelings would seem most appropriate to attribute to him?" The answer, of course, never came. But I achieved a perfect imitation by dint of continued practice. His gesture I made mine in the process. There are certain occasions, even today, in which I hear from my wife, "Why are you frowning like that?" And recollecting myself immediately, I realize that I often wear the mask of my dead father.

It is a curious fact that sights that were glanced at momentarily should linger forever, while others vanish in a trice that were contemplated intently for many years. The man who lifted me to the sight of my father's corpse lowered me after only a few seconds. The shawled women in the room looked at me with an insufferable, morbid inquisitiveness. I remained in the

room, by the door, not knowing what was expected of me but
firm in my resolve to show no emotion. At length the women's
glances left me, and the prayers resumed. Gradually in the course
of the religious service, perhaps as an effect of the hypnotic
intonation of the litanies, an indescribable heaviness came to
oppress me. It was the feeling of an absence, a hollowness, an
emptiness at the core of my being, that no created object could
possibly fulfill. And together with this feeling, tears welled up
in my eyes, and something like an inner sob clamored for release
in my bosom.

I discovered then, on the table by the door, among the coffee
cups and the snacks that sustained the women's uninterrupted
praying, the earthenware plate with the liquid hot-pepper sauce
that my father used to ingest. And without quite knowing what
I was doing, I took the large wooden spoon into my mouth and
guzzled a mouthful of the fiery compound. Two women took
me out of the room so that I could rinse and drink abundant
water, among exclamations of "The poor darling! He did not
know what was in that plate." And while abundant tears flowed
from my eyes, and grimacing contorted my face, I experienced
a strange satisfaction. I had contrived to burn the cry that was
forming in my throat, to flame it down to ashes before it became
viable. "Men don't cry" was the naïve code of masculinity that
my father voiced when he was alive, and I too young to take
my cue. Now that he was dead, I showed him that reflex
physiology, not a son's sorrow, was the cause of my tears.

It must have been twenty years later that we discarded the
last mementos of the mining company. There were stacks of
shareholders' certificates in fine, thick vellum. They were beau-
tifully decorated with a central logo that showed a hardy miner,

stripped to the waist, wearing a helmet with a flashlight on it and carrying a pick in his hands. The muscular torso, of classic Greek statuary proportions, and the determined look in his eyes, stood in sharp discrepancy with my recollection of the ragged peasant-miners who were actually intended to do the work. There were also yellowed newspaper clippings with large, bold-lettered captions that announced the discovery, by the district attorney's office, of a scheme of fraud, peculation, embezzlement, and other crimes. The name of my father, alas, figured prominently in these columns. I found also a letter that he had written to my mother during one of his trips. It described the progress made at the mine, and ended with a curious statement: "This time it is rags or riches for us." My mother commented, not without a touch of bitterness, when I read it to her, "As it turned out, it was rags for us, but not for him."

Let the sturdy moralist censure the profligate man who, having used up the family resources, leaves widow and orphans unprovided for. I, who saw the struggle, suspend my judgment and simply lay the facts before you. This man fought the telluric forces, and lost. To the formidable, awesome forces of nature, he replied with preposterous stratagems. Given the way he was, what else could he have done? Rash, improvident, unrealistic, and impractical: a dreamer: that is how he was.

Notes

Touch

1. The subject of pain in late fetal life and in small premature infants was recently discussed by K. J. S. Anand and P. R. Hickey in their monographic article "Pain and Its Effects in the Human Neonate and Fetus," *New England Journal of Medicine*, Vol. 317, no. 21 (November 19, 1987), 1321–1329. This article summarized the current medical opinion on the subject (201 references) and caused some commotion in nonmedical circles by drawing attention to ethical aspects of pain-producing medical procedures applied to an inherently defenseless population, namely infants and newborns. In the American magazine *Birth*, a mother reported with dismay how her baby had undergone a surgical operation with muscle relaxants and oxygen, but no anesthesia. See J. R. Lawson, letter to the editor, *Birth*, Vol. 13 (1986), 125–26. The indignation that ensued was not always well-informed, as discussed in an editorial in *The Lancet*, "Pain, Anesthesia, and Babies," Vol. 2 (September 5, 1987), 543–44.

2. Ludwig Wittgenstein, *Preliminary Studies for "Philosophical Investigations," Generally Known as the Blue and Brown Books* (New York: Harper & Row, 1965).

3. The late appearance of phantom limbs after amputation is mentioned by A. A. Bailey and F. P. Moersch in "Phantom Limbs," *Canadian Medical Association Journal*, Vol. 45 (1941), 37–42. Other works consulted were W. R. Henderson and G. E. Smyth, "Phantom Limbs," *Journal of Neurology,*

Neurosurgery and Psychiatry, Vol. 11 (1948), 88–112; and Karl Nielson, John E. Adams, and Yoshio Hosobuchi, "Phantom Limb Pain: Treatment with Dorsal Column Stimulation," *Journal of Neurosurgery*, Vol. 42 (March 1972), 301–7.

4. J. Prip-Møller, *Chinese Buddhist Monasteries. Their Plan and Function as a Setting for Buddhist Monastic Life* (Copenhagen: G.E.C. GADS Forlag, and London: Oxford University Press, 1937).

5. Quoted by R. R. Madden in *Phantasmata, or Illusions and Fanaticisms of Protean Forms Productive of Great Evils*, 2 vols. (London: T. C. Newby, 1857). See Vol. 1, Chapter 12, "The Flagellation Mania," 359–95.

6. Piero Ariotti, "Benedetto Castelli: Early Systematic Experiments and Theory of the Differential Absorption of Heat by Colors," *Isis*, Vol. 63, no. 21 (1972), 78–87.

7. Quoted by Bernard Cohen in "Franklin's Experiments in Heat Absorption as a Function of Color," *Isis*, Vol. 34, Part 5, no. 97 (1943), 404–6. According to Cohen, Franklin's observations were originally described in a letter to Mary Stevenson dated September 20, 1761, but were not published until years later, when they appeared in the introduction to the fourth edition of his celebrated work *Experiments and Observations on Electricity*.

8. Aldous Huxley, *The Doors of Perception* (London: Chatto & Windus, 1954).

9. Maurice Merleau-Ponty, *Phénoménologie de la Perception* (Paris: Gallimard, 1945), 245.

Hearing

1. The voices heard by Saint Augustine and Nero are described by John Aubrey (1626–1697), an interesting man and distinguished English writer born in Wiltshire and buried at Oxford in the Church of St. Mary Magdalene. He had a strong penchant for the "occult," was intimate with the men of science of his day, and compiled a curious record of supernatural phenomena, such as omens, dreams, apparitions, prophecies, and others. These are described with charming style in his *Miscellanies upon Various Subjects*, 4th ed. (London: John Russel Smith, 1857).

2. Auditory hallucinations accompany various forms of central nervous system disease. Although this topic is a highly technical one, the neurologist-writer Oliver Sacks has given a splendid exposition for the lay reader,

accompanied by scholarly references, in his popular book *The Man Who Mistook His Wife for a Hat, and Other Clinical Tales* (New York: Harper & Row, 1986). See, in particular, Chapter 15, entitled "Reminiscence." However, the phenomenon of musical hallucinations in "peripheral" forms of deafness was apparently ignored for a long time. See Elliott B. Ross, Paul B. Jossman, Benjamin Bell, Thomas Sabin, and Norman Geschwind, "Musical Hallucinations in Deafness," *Journal of the American Medical Association*, Vol. 231 (February 10, 1975), 620–22. This symptom had been recognized in Europe by H. Hécaen and P. Ropert, and reported in "Les Hallucinations auditives des otopathes," published in *Journal de Psychologie Normale et Pathologique* (Paris) Vol. 60 (1963), 293–324.

3. L. J. West, "A Clinical and Theoretical Overview of Hallucinatory Phenomena," in R. K. Siegel and L. J. West, eds., *Hallucination: Behavior, Experience and Theory* (New York: John Wiley, 1975), 301–2.

4. Dov Aizenberg, Bruria Schwartz, and Ilan Modai, "Musical Hallucinations, Acquired Deafness and Depression," *Journal of Nervous and Mental Diseases*, Vol. 174, no. 5 (May 1986), 309–11.

5. Jorge Luis Borges, *Siete Noches* (Mexico City: Fondo de Cultura Económica, 1981). A collection of a series of conferences given by Borges on different topics, one of them blindness.

6. Hein J. J. Wellens, Aart Vermeulen, and Dirk Durrer, "Ventricular Fibrillation Occurring on Arousal from Sleep by Auditory Stimuli," *Circulation*, Vol. 46 (1972), 661–65.

7. The quoted description of conjugal disharmony is owed to Xi-Jou Sheng, author of a novel that is considered a classic of Chinese literature, entitled *Exemplary Story of Matrimony*. I am unfortunately not aware of any published English-language translation, and gratefully acknowledge the assistance of my wife, Dr. Wei Hsueh, in translating the preface of this novel, where the mentioned description is to be found, from the Chinese text (Taiwan: Lian-Jin Publishers, 1986).

Smell

1. Etienne Bonnot de Condillac, *Traité des Sensations* (Paris: Charles Houel, 1789).

2. Max Delbrück, *Mind from Matter? An Essay in Evolutionary Epistemology* (Palo Alto: Blackwell Scientific Publications, 1986), 118.

3. *The Principal Works of Saint Jerome*, translated by the Hon. W. H. Freemantle, with the assistance of the Reverends G. Lewis and W. G. Martley (London: The Christian Literature Co., 1893). Reprinted in Vol. 6 of *A Select Library of Nicene and Post-Nicene Fathers of the Christian Church*, Second Series (New York: Charles Scribner's Sons, 1912). The quotation is from *Life of St. Hilarion* (28: 310), a work written by Jerome in the year 390, while at Bethlehem.

4. J. Collin de Plancy, *Dictionnaire Infernal* (Paris: Henri Plon, 1863). The sixth edition of this work was reprinted in 1980 by Slatkine Reprints, Geneva.

5. J. J. H. Ebers, "Hyperasthesie des Geruchssinnes als forensische Frage. Ein Diebes-Riecher," *Wochenschrift der Gerichtlichen öffentlichen Medizin*, Vol. 16 (1859), 278–96.

6. Georges Dumas, "L'odeur de sainteté," *La Revue de Paris*, 14ème Année (1907), 531–52. For another medical explanation of the odor of sanctity, see, "Odeur de sainteté et tumeur cérébrale," by A. Répond, in *Rev. méd. Suisse Romande* 46 (1926), 49–52.

7. Susan S. Schiffman, "Taste and Smell in Disease (Part 2)," *New England Journal of Medicine*, Vol. 308, no. 22 (June 2, 1983), 1337–43.

8. The anecdotes on malodorous chemists are quoted from the scholarly monograph by William McCarney, "Olfaction and Odors: An Osphresiological Essay" (New York: Springer-Verlag, 1968). Notwithstanding the use of the word "osphresiological" in the title, this encyclopedic work on olfaction is quite readable. It represents an honest attempt at summarizing the world's literature on human olfaction, with some attention to that of other species. It remains an indispensable reference for students of olfaction, although much has happened since its original publication.

9. Oliva Sabuco de Nantes Barrera, "Coloquio del Conocimiento de Sí Mismo," in Vol. 65 of *Biblioteca de Autores Españoles* (Madrid: M. Rivadeneyra, 1873), 350.

10. Quoted by P. Murray in *Le XIXe Siècle à travers les âges* (Paris: Denoël, 1984), 33.

11. B. Malinowski, *The Sexual Life of Savages in North-western Melanesia* (London: Routledge, 1929).

12. The "stereochemical" theory of olfaction has been championed by John E. Amoore. See his "Molecular Basis of Odor," Publication #773 of American Lecture Series (Springfield, Ill.: Charles C Thomas, 1970; also,

"Stereochemical Theory of Olfaction," *Nature*, Vol. 198 (1963), 271–72, and Vol. 199 (1963), 912–13.

13. J. T. Davies, "The Penetrating and Puncturing Theory of Odor," *J. Colloid Interface Sci.*, Vol. 29 (1969), 296.

14. Giacomo Leopardi *Pensieri di varia filosofia e di bella letteratura*, Vol. 3 (Florence: Félice Le Monnier, 1901), 219.

15. Sancti Pietri Damiani, "De Vita Sancti Romualdi Abbatis et Confessoris," in Vol. 2 of *Opera Omnia* (Bassano: Remondini, 1783), col. 741. Quoted by Piero Camporesi in *Le officine dei sensi* (Milan: Garzanti, 1985).

16. Theophrastus, "Concerning Odors," translated by Sir Arthur Hort in Vol. 2 of *Theophrastus' Inquiry into Plants* (New York: G. P. Putnam's Sons, 1916), 381.

17. R. Hamilton Wright, *The Science of Smell* (London: Allen and Unwin, 1964).

18. The following are accounts in the popular press of pertinent research: John Leo, "The Hidden Power of Body Odors: Studies Find That Male Pheromones Are Good for Women," *Time*, December 1, 1986; Terence Monmaney, with Susan Katz, "The Chemistry Between People: Are Our Bodies Affected by Another Person's Scent?", *Newsweek*, January 12, 1987; "Secrets of Sex: Does the Nose Know?" *Newsweek*, December 1, 1986; Stephen Budiansky, "Siren Song of the Pheromones; Chemicals in Males' Sweat Can Increase the Chance of Pregnancy," *U.S. News & World Report*, December 1, 1986.

19. Television program entitled "Innovation," written by Jill Peters and aired by PBS in Chicago on September 6, 1987.

Sight

1. Roland Barthes, *Empire of Signs*, translated by Richard Howard (New York: Farrar, Straus & Giroux, 1982), 99–102.

2. Lin Cheng-Hin, "Oriental Blepharoplasty: A Critical Review of Technique and Potential Hazards," *Annals of Plastic Surgery*, Vol. 7 (November 1981), 362–74.

3. Joseph DiLeo, M.D., *Interpreting Children's Drawings* (New York: Brunner/Mazel Publishers, 1983), 115–16.

4. Charles Singer, "A Study in Early Renaissance Anatomy, with a Text:

The *Anothomia* of Hieronymo Manfredi (1940)," in *Studies in the History and Method of Science*, C. Singer, ed. (London: William Dawson & Sons, 1955), 118–22.

5. Francis Bacon, "Of Envy," in *Essays* (New York: Walter J. Black, 1942), 32.

6. The "evil eye" has been the subject of considerable scholarly work. For an English-language book of relatively recent printing, see Edward S. Gifford, *The Evil Eye—Studies in the Folklore of Vision* (New York: Macmillan, 1958). A well-written article by an American ophthalmologist, and a good source of references, is *"Oculus fascinus,"* by Benjamin L. Gordon, in *Archives of Ophthalmology*, Vol. 17 (1937), 291–319. A comprehensive two-volume German treatise also exists, although it is less easily available: S. Seligman, *Der Böse Blick* (Berlin: Herman Barsdorf Verlag, 1910).

7. Théophile Gautier, "Jettatura," in *Récits Fantastiques* (Paris: Flammarion, 1981), 379–474.

8. Jerome T. Pearlman, George L. Adams, and Sherwin H. Sloan, eds., *Psychiatric Problems in Ophthalmology* (Springfield, Ill.: Charles C Thomas, 1977).

9. Phyllis Greenacre, "Eye Motif in Delusion and Fantasy," *American Journal of Psychiatry*, Vol. 5 (1926), 553–79.

10. Ch. Lasègue, *Les exhibitionnistes*, Union Médicale (Paris), Series 3, no. 50 (May 1, 1877), 710–14.

11. Irvin D. Yalom, "Aggression and Forbiddenness in Voyeurism," *Archives of General Psychiatry*, Vol. 3 (September 1960), 305–19.

12. Marc E. Hollender, Winston C. Brown, and H. B. Roback, "General Exhibitionism in Women," *American Journal of Psychiatry*, Vol. 134, no. 4 (April 1977), 436–38.

13. Milton Eber, "Exhibitionism or Narcissism?" (editorial), *American Journal of Psychiatry*, Vol. 134, no. 9 (September 1977), 1053.